God
Sex
Food

A Guide to Diet and
Exercise Honoring God

ENJOY !

Dr. Karl N. Kaluza

Karl

INTELLECTUALLY HONEST PUBLISHING, LLC

Lake Oswego, Oregon

<u>God</u>
<u>Sex</u>
<u>Food</u>

Printed in the United States of America
First Printing, 2013

ISBN: 0615901026
ISBN 13: 978-0-615-90102-2

Intellectually Honest Publishing, LLC
569 6th St.
Lake Oswego, Oregon 97034

USA

*"Do you not know that your bodies
are temples of the Holy Spirit, who is in you,
whom you have received from God?
You are not your own; you were bought at a price.
Therefore honor God with your bodies."*

1 Corinthians 6:19-20

Table of Contents:

Forward ·· vii

Chapter 1 Repentance ·····································1

Chapter 2 Science Lesson #1 – Artificial Sweeteners ··········5

Chapter 3 Searching for God ······························15

Chapter 4 Science Lesson #2 – Why Food is Like Sex ·······19

Chapter 5 Higher Education···························· 25

Chapter 6 Science Lesson #3 – Understanding Your
Metabolism – The Old Grey Mare She
Ain't What She Used to Be····················29

Chapter 7 Medical School ····························· 33

Chapter 8 Science Lesson #4 – Diet Pills and Shots········· 41

Chapter 9 The Jesus Problem ···························· 49

Chapter 10 Science Lesson #5 – Medical Causes of a Slow
Metabolism Exist – Make Sure You
Don't Have One ································57

Chapter 11 Trying on Jesus to See How He Fits ············· 65

Chapter 12 Science Lesson #6 – Fourth Grade Math and
Department Store Mirrors····················· 69

Chapter 13 A Word from Our Sponsor ····················· 77

Chapter 14 Science Lesson # 7 – Food Labels and Marketing··· 81

Chapter 15 And Then I Learned I Am a Sinner ············· 95

Chapter 16 Science Lesson #8 – The Glycemic Index ········ 103

Chapter 17 Idolatry of Food and the Destruction of the Temple ···111

Chapter 18 Science Lesson #9 – The Sports Psychology of
Eating ······································· 119

Chapter 19 A Word on Guilt ··························· 125

Chapter 20 Science Lesson # 10 – A Summary On a
Healthy Temple:····························· 129

Chapter 21 A Benediction ····························· 135

Forward:

"The word of the Lord came to Jonah son of Ammatia: "Go to the city of Nineveh and preach against it, because its wickedness has come up before me." But Jonah ran away from the Lord and headed for Tarshish." Jonah 1:1-3*

The Lord called me to write this book long before I started it. Like Jonah, I ran away from my assignment. Like Jonah, I did not want to do what God was asking of me. I did not run away from my home outside of Portland, Oregon. Instead, for years, I just tried to ignore His call. But that is the middle of the story. Let me start at the beginning.

Chapter: 1

Repentance

"And Jesus answered them, "Those who are well have no need of a physician, but those who are sick. I have not come to call the righteous but sinners to repentance."' Mark 2:7

My father struck me once. Although it was a long time ago I still remember it clearly. It felt like being hit in the face with a two-by-four. He was a big and powerful man, a former heavyweight wrestler and state champion football player. After the blow I felt stunned. Like a concussion. I have had a lot of concussions so I would know.

I was 18 at the time and full of testosterone and full of myself. I was in very good shape from exercising three hours a day including a minimum of one hour of weight lifting. My dad was fat, and I was letting him know it. "Dad, I thought you were an athlete. What happened to you?" He looked me in the eye until he had my full attention. And then he unloaded on me. "Before you make too much fun of me, you should take a look close look at your family tree", he said. At first I chortled. And then, as I realized the full gravity of what he had hit me with, I was struck dazed and mute.

My mind raced through the family. Fat, fat, fat, fat, fat...every member of my family, with the exception of my scrawny younger sister, was obese. I mean all of them. Grandparents, check. Every aunt, check. Every uncle, check. Mom, check. Dad, check. I saw my fate. And I did not like it.

I have always been a good problem solver, and I clearly had a problem. I started by looking to the common features of my family.

Everyone was obese. Everyone, with the exception of Uncle Mike, ate a balanced diet. Mike loved hot chocolate made with two packets of cocoa instead of the typical one packet, and was well-known for eating Twinkies. But, everyone else typically had all of the food groups with their meals. Many exercised. I needed to identify a common theme or problem shared by my family that I personally could avoid or change. My problem solving was not bearing any fruit. It was bearing only despair. Perhaps I needed to look to a counterexample. I tried to think of a distant relative who was not fat. I had no luck. I decided to cast a larger net to include other adults.

Most of my friend's parents were overweight as well, but not all. I concentrated on the non-fat counterexamples. One had a touchy stomach and could not eat much. Another ran 5 miles every day at 5am. Another went rowing a few times a week, drank tea often, and ate rarely. Another, the most attractive mom of the bunch, was known for never having been seen eating. Ever. Were there any lessons here for me? Yes. But I did not like them.

I guessed that running five miles a day for the rest of my life would probably work, but I did not care that much for running. It conjured butterflies in my stomach with images of an upset coach bringing his whistle to his lips and letting loose a shrill blow, followed shortly by, "ON THE LINE," followed shortly by me gasping for air and hoping someone else would give out before me. Ideally the coach would relent, but another teammate throwing up on the field usually made the running come to a halt as well. I was happy to run while chasing a ball or while at play, but running just for running was a punishment. Some masochists may like the idea of being punished for the rest of their life. Do not count me among them.

I likewise guessed that eating like a bird would probably work. The problem here was that these thin bird-like people obviously did not like food the way I like food. I have always liked food: The yeasty smell of baking bread, the sizzle of an egg fried crisp at the edges but soft in the middle, the evolving texture as you work your way from the outside to the center of a cinnamon roll, the stark contrast between a grocery store tomato and those grown by my grandmother, the way smoked fish can be both dry and moist at the same time, picking through three different aromas and six different flavors in one sip of wine, timing how long after the last sliver of dark chocolate has melted in your mouth you can still clearly taste the chocolate, and even some of the subtle citrus, the first bite of a honey-crisp apple, peaches that seem to contain more juice than is physically possible in a fruit of that size, pizza cooked in a scorching hot wood oven with just a bit too much char on the crust, homemade ice cream. I could go on. I still had a problem.

Maybe science could help. I was planning to follow my father's footsteps to medical school. I decided I would pay more attention to exercise, nutrition, and genetics along the way and look for a more evolved answer.

Chapter: 2

Science Lesson #1 –
Artificial Sweeteners

"A false balance is an abomination to the Lord, but a just weight is his delight. When pride comes, then comes disgrace, but with the humble is wisdom." Proverbs 11:1-2

A glass of Coca-Cola tastes good. Soda is even better poured over nugget ice. Not everyone is familiar with nugget ice. Nugget ice used to be more common. It is the type of ice that looks like small pellets of highly compressed snow. The Coke seeps into the center of these nuggets creating a glass filled with mini Coke snow-cones. It is probably not the type of ice you would pick for mating with scotch, but pairing with Coke is pure symbiosis.

You have seen the soda fountain at the restaurant or convenience store. Have you noticed that the heaviest people are the most likely to be drinking the diet soda? You can do your own survey of this at the grocery store as well. Note who has the case of diet soda in their cart. Give some attention to who is choosing the sugar free ice-cream. There may be a counter-example or two at first, but if you collect enough of your own data you will notice a trend that sugar free means more likely to be fat. I thought it was a choice people were making because of their weight, but that may not be the whole story. Let's start with rats.

When rats are in a cage it is possible to know all of the calories they eat by counting the number of pellets and volume of liquid they consume. It is also easy to weigh them. Testing done at Purdue University and released in the *Journal of Neuroscience* found that rats fed artificial sweetener gained more weight than rats fed a sugary diet.

The extra weight gain was partially accounted for by these rats eating more pellets. Unfortunately, the rats lack the communication skills to tell us why they ate more pellets. The assumption is that they were hungrier than the other group. But, the extra pellets alone did not account for all of the weight gain. This group gained more weight than the extra pellets could produce. This is harder to explain. There are two possibilities. It is possible the artificial sweetener rats moved less and thus burned fewer calories. The other option is that their metabolic rate was slowed by their diet and they thus burned fewer calories.

This metabolic idea appears to be part of the answer. When you heat your home it takes energy to make the heat. The higher you set the thermostat the more gas or electricity you have to pay for. If you heat with wood, you have to add more logs to the fire if you want it to be hotter. Bodies are no different. You have to burn more calories to make a body warmer. The rats eating the artificial sweetener had lower body temperatures, thus implying a decrease in their calorie burn (metabolism).

I am not a rat, so perhaps I don't care very much if artificial sweetener makes rats fat. But, I would care if it also makes people fat. Let's travel to Framingham, Massachusetts. Since 1948 data has been collected on the people of Framingham. The Framingham study includes what people eat, drink, and smoke. It includes their weight, cholesterol levels, and blood pressures. Study of this population is why we know that smoking increases the risk of heart attacks and aspirin decreases the risk. The people of this town have been followed very closely for over 60 years and the data collection started before the first artificial sweetener (saccharin) was invented in 1950.

The Framingham data released by the American Heart Association's journal *Circulation* in 2007 shows distressing results. People who use artificial sweeteners have a 50% higher risk of being fat, having high cholesterol, having high blood pressure, and also of having diabetes. Fifty percent is significant. I cannot name another food, drink, or activity associated with such high odds. The association between smoking and lung cancer is well known. But, only 20% of lifelong heavy smokers will get lung cancer. Less than 50% of children who fall out of fourth story windows die. Only 2% of allied troops died on D-day. Again, increasing odds 50% is significant.

When I first read the odds associated with the diet soda I thought to myself, "Well, sure there is a link, but the link is that the people drinking the soda are overweight. It is the weight causing both the diet soda use and the extra diabetes and high blood pressure and high cholesterol." Well, it turns out that things like total calorie intake, saturated fat intake, trans-fat intake, and sedentary lifestyle were taken into account by the researchers. And the 50% increase still held true.

Now, this does not prove that diet soda is the culprit. There may be some other association that explains the marked rise in disease incidence. Perhaps people that consume artificial sweeteners are also participating in another behavior that is the true root of the problem. As the Framingham data was controlled for variables known to be associated with increased risk, this root would be of profound importance to know about. For instance, what if diet soda drinkers were also more likely to snack after midnight, and it is really the nocturnal feeding that is the cause of the problem? All concentration should then be moved from the artificial sweeteners to locking up the kitchen after bedtime.

Another alternative is that there is something about the people otherwise pre-disposed to these illnesses that causes them to be drawn to the diet products. For instance, perhaps listening to country music causes both the diabetes and the craving for the artificial sweeteners. The artificial sweetener is thus an effect rather than the cause. Maybe looking at other studies on artificial sweeteners will be enlightening.

If we go back to an era of neon, big hair, and trickle-down economics there is a large study available. The *Journal of Preventive Medicine* in 1986 released a prospective study of 78,000 women including artificial sweetener data. This study showed a statistically significant increase in weight in the artificial sweetener users. The authors specifically comment that the weight gain was "not explicable by differences in food consumption patterns." Apparently similar to the Purdue rats, the women in this study gained weight that could not be accounted for simply by an increase in food or calorie intake. Again, this study does not prove causation. But, it is another 78,000 data points.

Another study including artificial sweetener data was released in 2008 in the journal *Obesity*. It studied 5,158 adults in Texas over the span of nine years looking at factors which influence obesity. Similar to the Framingham data, this study showed an increased risk of developing obesity in artificial sweetener users. The more artificial sweetener that people consumed the more weight they gained. There was a dose dependent rise in body mass index with artificial sweetener use. In fact, the participants that consumed twenty-one or more servings per week had a doubling of risk of developing obesity.

The ARIC (Atherosclerosis Risk in Communities) study began in 1987 to look at risk factors for diabetes, high cholesterol, and obesity. Released in 2008 in the American Heart Association's journal *Circulation*, this was a prospective study of almost 10,000 Americans from ages 45 to 64. The goal of this study was to look at the role of diet in the development of metabolic syndrome. Metabolic syndrome is the combination of obesity, high blood pressure, high cholesterol, and/or high blood sugar. The presence of metabolic syndrome significantly increases the risk of heart attacks, strokes, and diabetes. Even if it did not increase the risk of a heart attack it still sounds unpleasant to me anyway.

The study results were adjusted for factors such as age, sex, race, study site, education level, caloric intake, smoking, and exercise. The study results showed very strong risk increase in metabolic syndrome with fried foods and meats such as hot dogs. Study designers had hypothesized that fruits and vegetables and whole grains would be protective against developing metabolic syndrome and were surprised to find that this was not the case.

They were also surprised to find that contrary to hypothesis, juice and sugar-sweetened soda were not associated with development of metabolic syndrome.

The only food group that was shown to be protective against metabolic syndrome was dairy which is consistent with other literature on the topic. The food most strongly associated with development of metabolic syndrome was diet soda. The diet soda finding was not hypothesized at study design, but the authors note that it is consistent with the Framingham data and deserves further study. The MESA (Multi-Ethnic Study of Atherosclerosis) study did just that.

The MESA study released in *Diabetes Care* in 2009 sought to specifically look at the role of diet soda in the incidence of developing diabetes and metabolic syndrome "while taking into consideration multiple lifestyle confounders." The study involved almost 7000 adults spread all around the United States and spanned from the years 2000 to 2007. Race, age, sex, location, food intake, education, exercise, smoking, vitamin use, and a variety of specific food intake patterns such as whole grain intake, fruit and vegetable intake, sugar sweetened soda intake, saturated fat intake, and coffee intake were all taken into consideration. The study was further adjusted for baseline waist circumference, BMI (body mass index: a measure of weight relative to height), body weight, and changes in all of these measures over time.

The results of this study show a 36% increased risk of developing metabolic syndrome in diet soda consumers. Looking further at the confounders, the results could not be explained by demographic or geographic consideration. Nor could they be explained by caloric intake, food type intake, or nutrient or vitamin intake.

The MESA data for diabetes risk was even greater than that seen in the Framingham study. Diet soda drinkers were found to develop diabetes 67% more than non-drinkers. With regard to diabetes development, none of the confounders were found to be associated with this increased risk. The authors again are careful to state that there may be some unknown confounder playing a secret role.

The weight gain seen in artificial sweetener users is seen in the elderly as well. A portion of a longitudinal aging study was presented by University of Texas researchers at the 2011 meeting of the American Diabetes Association. Elderly diet soda drinkers had an increase in waist circumference 500% greater than diet soda abstainers over the course of this long-running study. No other food or drink was found to be even close to such a great factor.

If we delve deeper into diabetes specifically, there is some artificial sweeter data to look at there as well. Diabetics who use artificial sweeteners (commonly recommended by American Diabetes Association nutritionists) actually have worse diabetic control than non-users. This is definitely true amongst my patients and the effect seems dose dependent where the more artificial sweetener consumed, the higher the average blood sugar. I think a part of this is from the personality of the user and part from the sweetener itself. It may be that people trying to cheat by using artificial sweeteners are also more likely to cheat in other aspects of their diet.

What about factors other than fatness? A 2010 study in the *American Journal of Clinical Nutrition* studied almost 60,000 pregnant women to look at how diet affects pregnancy. The study showed that artificial sweetener use was associated with increased risk of pre-term delivery in both overweight and normal weight women. The increase in risk was again striking. Women drinking one or more diet sodas a day had a 38% increased risk of delivering before 37 weeks (pre-term). Women drinking four or more diet sodas a day were 78% more likely than non-diet soda drinkers to have a pre-term delivery. There was no effect seen with consumption of sugar-sweetened soda.

Starting in 1976, 250,000 female nurses have participated in The Nurses' Health Study which has been a source of significant and new information on women's health. For instance, it is out of this study that use of hormone replacement was found to be linked to a higher risk of breast cancer. In 2009 it was released that consumption of diet soda doubles the risk of kidney failure. This doubling of risk was still true when other variables that tend to affect kidney function such as diabetes, obesity, and high blood pressure were taken into account. As only women were studied, it is unknown if this is true of men.

Researchers at Columbia University found that diet soda was also a risk factor for vascular events with daily users suffering 43% more strokes and heart attacks than non-users. The study was controlled for known risk factors such as high blood pressure, diabetes, and obesity. The increased risk was not seen in regular soda drinkers.

Now, with all of this data to suggest that perhaps it is inadvisable to drink diet soda, you may think that it would be a simple thing to suggest as a behavior change to my patients. In some cases it is. In many cases it causes significant anger. People have placed belief in something. In this case it is perhaps belief in scientific advancement which will ultimately lead to societal improvement or self-improvement. Perhaps the belief is that the artificial sweetener is good for you...or at least not as bad as whatever else you may eat and drink. It is unpleasant to find that your beliefs are placed in something false. Some patients simply persist in a state of chronic denial. Others go through an anger stage. As I am typically the only other person in the room, the anger is often directed at me.

I am much more delighted to have an angry response or an inquisitive one than an apathetic response. I can often tell in the subtle glazing of my patient's eyes that they are not interested in hearing more on this topic. They either don't want to change their behavior, or more likely, they don't want to have to change their belief. Angry and even defiant questioning, however, I find encouraging. It implies that the patient cares. I can use that caring to help to guide them to greater vitality.

I have found the analogy of smoking to be helpful. I have a well-educated patient population. The majority doesn't smoke and reviles the idea of it. They also know I don't smoke. I then explain that, knowing what I know, I would rather smoke a cigarette than drink a can of diet soda. Remember, I am vain regarding my weight. I know that smoking can lead to lung cancer (20% of life-long smokers) and emphysema. I also know that smoking is associated with weight loss. I will take the slim waist and a 20% chance of lung cancer over a 50% chance of diabetes and obesity any day. And then my patient sees that I am not joking about the smoking. Since they know I would not dream of smoking cigarettes, the gravity of my words seems to sink in.

There is power in knowledge. Use this empowering knowledge of artificial sweeteners to your advantage. A list of artificial and non-nutritive sweeteners can be found in Afterward A at the end of the book.

Chapter: 3

Searching for God

"Now hope that is seen is not hope. For who hopes for what he sees?" Romans 8:24

My favorite commercial of all time stars two bighorn sheep butting heads. I do not recall what the commercial advertised, but I will never forget the massive scrotum of the sheep on the right side of the screen. The scrotum swings back and forth at least one foot as the horns of the rams collide. I still cannot believe the commercial made the cut past the FCC.

While I am amused by that sheep with the big balls, I do not think very highly of sheep in general. They have a reputation for being loud, malodorous, and dumb. It seems to me that being a sheep with God or Jesus as the shepherd may not be all that appealing. But let me back up a few years.

The moment came near the end of high school. I had been raised lovingly in the church. My family attended services together most Sundays. I went to Bible study most Sundays. We prayed before each dinner. But when my faith came under a little fire, I found it was not very strong.

In my church there was a formal ceremonial declaration of faith made by young adults. People were run through this ceremony as a class and so all of my friends with whom I had been attending Sunday school would be making this public declaration of faith with me. Except for Ryan.

Ryan confided in me one day that he was not going to go through with it. He stated simply that he was not sure he believed in God, and that if he was not sure then he was not going to say otherwise, especially in public. I was somewhat shocked. Ryan was not a rebel. He was a well-respected leader at school and was known for public acts of morality such as drinking milk at parties instead of beer. I tried to talk him out of it. "What about your parents? They will be devastated," I said. Ryan said he did not care.

Now, I know he did care, for he was a respectful son. What he really meant was that he cared more about being true to himself than he cared about his parents feelings. This got me to thinking.

What did I believe? I found, unfortunately, I was not sure. All of what I knew about God and scripture I had been fed by my parents and the church. I was worldly enough to realize that neither was an absolute authority. Anyone who has parents knows this about them. History was sufficient to prove that the church was a suspect authority figure. Did God exist? What was the meaning of life? I decided to look for such answers.

I followed through with my public proclamation of faith, not for me, but to honor my parents. In weighing being true to my own beliefs and disappointing my parents, it was an easy decision at the time to make mom and dad happy. I figured I would sort things out later. And what better place than the halls of an academic institution? I picked my college because they had the highest acceptance rate to medical school. It was a very small private liberal arts university in Washington State called The University of Puget Sound. The school just happened to have a very good philosophy program. I had long ago decided my pre-med major, now I had my minor.

Chapter: 4

Science Lesson #2 –
Why Food is Like Sex

"Be fruitful and multiply…." Genesis 1:28

Sex, drugs, music, love, sports, drinking, and eating are all sources of pleasure. There is a common feature of all of these pleasurable activities. They cause neurotransmitter release in the brain. And these brain chemicals are good stuff.

" It's like this fuzzy warm tingle that starts in my toes. When my toes get into it, I know it's there. After that it feels like I'm coasting in this super sensitive and almost overwhelming state where my whole body is simultaneously tense and relaxed (in reality I know it's pretty tense, but a good tense). My breathing is always what signifies the orgasm is arriving. My breathing starts feeling like I just ran a race – like my lungs are tired.

Then the actual orgasm starts down below and travels in
a wave all the way up to my head. I wouldn't describe it
as an explosion, though I've heard that before. It's more
like a powerful wave of blankness. The orgasm itself
feels good, but not as good as the before and after stages
because it's kind of like being knocked out for a bit.
Then I come-to (so to speak) in what has to be the
most relaxed and happy state ever. After I orgasm it's
like my lungs feel happy, as though I've been
breathing a lot of brisk fresh air."
-anonymous

Sexual activity and orgasm are associated with the release of significant amounts of these brain chemicals: serotonin, oxytocin, epinephrine, norepinephrine, and dopamine all play a role in sexual arousal and orgasm. Without these neurotransmitter chemicals working behind the scenes, there is no erection, no vaginal lubrication, and no orgasm.

A 2003 article in *The Journal of Neuroscience* looked at the neurotransmitter dopamine in connection with orgasm using PET scanning (a scan which measures brain use). Orgasm was as potent as heroin in causing dopamine release. The orgasm dopamine release is further established by the effect of orgasm on restless leg syndrome. This syndrome is an unpleasant urge to move the legs while at rest. It is associated with dopamine transport problems. Drugs that improve dopamine transport (Parkinson's medications) relieve this unpleasant urge. As reported in *Sleep Medicine* in 2011, orgasm improves restless legs too.

Street drugs cause a direct release of neurotransmitters as their mechanism of action. Different drugs work on different neurotransmitters. Cocaine releases dopamine and adrenaline resulting in turbocharged euphoria. Ecstasy releases serotonin resulting in calm cool euphoria. Heroin and the other narcotics release dopamine and mimic the body's own endorphin, stimulating a painless calm euphoria. The THC in marijuana binds to the body's anandamide neurotransmitter receptor and turns it on, resulting in a calm euphoria with a heightening of the senses and an effect on mood, memory, appetite, and pain.

What about the brain research with regard to cognitive activities of pleasure? A recent article in *Nature Neuroscience* proved that music which is perceived as pleasurable stimulates dopamine release from the brain. Perhaps this can help to explain the great lengths and costs that music lovers will go to in order to get a good fix.

Food, too, evokes a neurotransmitter response for pleasure. Serotonin and dopamine are both involved with certain foods seeming to have a greater effect than others. For instance, dark chocolate raises serotonin levels significantly. Dark chocolate, while less potent, is otherwise difficult to distinguish from orgasm with regard to the effect on the brain. No wonder we like chocolate.

As the experiences that create these good neurotransmitter responses are rewarding, the behavior that underlies the neurotransmitter response is encouraged. This reward response is the most basic behavioral training system. Dog sits and dog gets a cookie. Dog learns that sitting is rewarding. Therefore, dog sits when asked. As humans, we like to think we are more advanced than other animals. Looking to see what happens when the reward is removed will help to see if this advancement is true.

Recall that the active drug in marijuana, THC, increases appetite as part of binding to the neurotransmitter receptor. Perhaps it would be useful to block this receptor with weight loss as the intended goal. Just such a drug was created in 1994 called rimonabant (Acomplia). When taken daily, this THC receptor blocker significantly decreased weight, waist circumference, insulin levels, and cholesterol levels. A medication called naloxone blocks the euphoric effect of opiates. This is quite useful in the setting of a heroin overdose where the suppression of breathing and loss of consciousness are immediately reversed by the neurotransmitter receptor blocker. Interestingly, this same opiate receptor has an effect on the behavior of unnaturally tan people. You may know someone that goes to the tanning bed too much and appears possibly addicted to tanning. Naloxone removes the pleasure these people experience with tanning and significantly reduces tanning behavior. Oh, and it decreases narcotic abuse as well.

All of this brain chemistry mumbo-jumbo is important because it helps to explain what drives our behavior. We are designed to seek pleasure and avoid pain. Having looked at some sources of pleasure, it is no great stretch of the mind to see that there are ways to use these pleasure sources that are not beneficial. Drug abuse, sexual perversion, gluttony, and financial irresponsibility are all possible outcomes of seeking after these happy neurotransmitters. But that is only half the story.

Some poor decisions can come from simple pleasure seeking. Perhaps initially the drug addict was just looking for a good time. And the drug did feel very good. But not anymore. Initially to get the drugs you can just pay for them. But after some time the money is gone. Then you have to start selling things. Your stereo. Your TV. Your car. Your rent or mortgage payment. Your body. If there are no buyers or no stuff left then it is time to start stealing. With the stealing comes destruction of not only the self but also the surrounding world. Prostitution, thievery, and destruction are painful. They are just not as painful as something else.

There are a couple of options that would explain a life of pain so great that being a hopeless addict is preferable. The easiest answer is that the withdrawal from the drugs is so unpleasant and unrelenting that everything and everyone must be sacrificed to make the pain stop. In the moment, more of the drugs is the only thing that will work. The other source of pain is a little sadder to me. It is possible that the real life of the addict is so painful that the stupor of the drug is better.

Instead of drug abuse, what about abuse of another source of pleasure? What causes us to eat in ways that are unhealthy? Like with drugs, some harmful eating comes from simple pleasure seeking. Tillamook mint chip ice cream is hard for me to resist, even if I am full and don't need any more food. But there are other psychologies that play a role with eating.

I am competitive. I know it. My wife knows it. My kids know it. My friends know it. A small part of this comes from the enjoyment of winning. Truthfully however, a larger part comes from not wanting to lose. The winning produces the good neurotransmitters, but losing produces pain. And avoiding that pain is really what drives my competitive nature.

Now take an example of my overweight patient Samantha. Samantha has high cholesterol, high waist circumference, high blood sugar, and presents for an annual physical. She has weighed around 200lb since the birth of her last child. She has tried a number of diets which led to temporary weight loss over the course of her life but has never stuck with one very long. I give Samantha counsel on how to eat better and how to exercise. It is a plan that will work if she can stick to it. I want to see her back in two weeks to see how she is doing.

Two weeks later Samantha shows up having gained four pounds. Why? Because, like me, she hates to lose. The pain of failure that she has experienced with all (100%) of her prior trials at weight loss is real. She does not want to experience this pain again. The most assured way to avoid this is to not try. If Samantha does not try, she can't be disappointed in herself. She gets to avoid the pain of failure. Similar psychology is present in most forms of self-destructive behavior.

The point of all of this talk on neurotransmitters is to admit that they are driving some of our behavior. Topping off your pleasure tank only with food, or using food to compensate for sad or distressing feelings does work. But, there is a price to pay. Using food as this type of tool leads to eating more calories than the body needs. The brain will tell you to keep eating as it desires the pleasure, even if the pleasure is harmful in other ways. Continued use despite adverse consequences is the definition of addiction.

There will be little will for change in behavior until there is insight that there is a problem. That is true of all forms of harmful behavior. Step one then is to ask yourself, or your doctor, or God, or someone who will not lie to you if there is a problem. You probably already know there is a problem. The next step is to look for the cause. Are you fueling for pleasure? Are you fueling to avoid pain? Are you behaving as an addict with continued use despite adverse consequences? Without this type of insight you can be really, really smart, but your good judgment will be impaired. To work, judgment needs insight.

Chapter: 5

Higher Education

"Wisdom is supreme. Therefore get wisdom." Proverbs 4:7

I had no intention of experiencing the world while in college. My single goal was to get into medical school. But, along the way, if some fun happened to come my way, that would be OK with me. On the first Friday night of school there was an off-campus party thrown by one of the fraternities. My new acquaintance from upstairs, Matt, insisted that I go to this party. Matt steered us through the neighborhood. Matt got us past the front door. Matt led us past the dancing girls to the back of the kitchen where the keg of beer sat. Matt procured two beers and handed one to me. It was my first beer. I was uneasy with all of this. Until I had my first sip. Time slowed. I still remember very clearly thinking, "Oh, this is good. Why have I not been drinking this my whole life?" Some people develop a taste for beer. For me it was love at first sip.

Throughout college I maintained a constant focus on my goal of gaining entry to medical school. I earned excellent grades. Though I had to study more than the business majors, I was blessed to have to study much less than the typical science major. My medical school top priority was in good form. But, my secondary priority, to learn the meaning of life through the study of philosophy and religion, had developed some competition: Beer, Girls, and Sports.

I played a variety of sports in high school, but in college I focused on lacrosse. Lacrosse is a fast-paced and violent game. I liked the pace and loved the violence. I spent plenty of time in the penalty box as a result of this. There is a strong lacrosse tradition of beer drinking after games. When you scored your first goal the team had a tradition: you were thrust on a rooftop above the post-game party and encouraged to drink beer while the rest of the party with beers raised in salute sang to you over and over "He's happy, he's jolly, he'll eat shit by golly."

I was reading Plato, Aristotle, and Nietzsche for class, but it seemed to me that perhaps the meaning of life was no more complicated than the right mix of sports, beer, and girls. I did my best to partake in as large of a quantity of each as my studies of the thoughts of dead men would allow. And it was fantastic few years. Then Hope left me.

The entrance exam for medical school is called the medical college admissions test or MCAT. It is the single most defining and important measure of quality for medical school admission. I had been studying for this test for years. A few days before the big test, the phone rang. It was Hope. She wanted to break up.

We'd been dating for almost four years and I loved her. We were best friends. I put my trust in her. I trusted her more than

26

anyone else in my life. I planned to marry her after college. It was one of the great shocks of my life.

I leapt head first into the first stage of grieving known as denial. I climbed into bed and tried to make it go away. But, recall, I am a problem solver. So, I wandered into the bargaining stage of grieving. I wanted to fly to Wisconsin to convince her she was making a mistake. She said no. I almost went anyway, but I had a test standing in my way. I had some friends at her school so I called them for an inside scoop. They were kind and caring and loving. But, they confirmed there had been another man in her bed. That would steer many people into the anger stage of grief, but I remained in the bargaining stage. I thought I would finish my test, and then deal with things in Wisconsin. But, truth be told, I was not doing well.

I could not eat. I skipped classes. I no-showed for parties. I skipped practices. I mostly just lay in bed and cried. I cried until I was too dry to make tears, then I just blubbered away with a dry throat. My friend and longtime roommate, Colby, had been doing what he knew to try in this situation by bringing food that I would not eat and water I would not drink. Eventually he either got frustrated with me or scared for me and called in backup. My mom lived 3.5 hours away. She arrived in three hours flat after Colby called her.

As far as losing innocence, I had it pretty easy compared to most. But, it was still very hard in the moment. Seeing the unconditional love in my mother's eyes was both a good reminder of what love should look like and a painful contrast to lost conditional love. But, feeling loved in that moment was something I needed. I think of that as the defining triumph of my mother's love for her son. I realize there may have been harder moments for her, but that is when I needed someone most, and she was there with open arms.

Maybe girls were not the meaning of life. They are more fun than playing with fire, but also much more painful than getting burned. I have had many injuries including tooth extractions, concussions, lacerations, blood poisoning, busted ankle, broken hand, busted fingers, broken nose, busted ribs, and a collapsed lung. All added together, they did not hurt as much as the heartache from a girl. Maybe beer and sports were still safe.

Chapter: 6

Science Lesson #3 – Understanding Your Metabolism – The Old Grey Mare She Ain't What She Used to Be

"For the living know they will die; but the dead do not know anything, nor have they any longer a reward, for their memory is forgotten." Ecclesiastes 9:5

I commonly bring up the issue of weight in my office. Obesity increases risk for infections, more days missed from work, high cholesterol, diabetes, heart disease, sleep apnea, etc. Allow me to introduce Joe.

At his wife's insistence, 40 year-old Joe came to see me for a physical. Joe had high cholesterol, high blood pressure, and high blood sugar. Joe, successful and handsome, oozes confidence. He played football in high school and still works out now. Joe is six feet tall and weighs 235 pounds. At graduation from high school was six feet tall and 210 pounds. But Joe was stronger playing football than he is now. Some of his weight has moved from his muscles to his belly. If he looks at himself in the mirror face-to-face then he looks pretty good. From the side however, a gut pooches forth.

Joe's lab results and vital signs perplexed him. As we get to the discussion of ways to fix what is causing these abnormalities Joe gives me the stink eye when I suggest weight loss. He says, "Doc, I eat the same as I always have, and I work out every day."

So we travel back in time. I ask, "What did you weigh when you graduated high school?" and, "Were you stronger then or now?" and, "Have you gotten any taller?" The point of this questioning is to lead Joe to the conclusion that at the same height, and weaker, then the extra weight is fat weight. This takes more time with some patients than with others. On top of the 25 pounds that the superficial math would suggest, there is an additional fat weight accounted for by the decreased strength. It is possible that Joe is carrying 10+ pounds less lean muscle so that the total fat weight gain since graduation is really 35 pounds or more.

Now, I believe Joe that he is exercising and not eating any differently than he has in the past. And that is exactly his problem.

Your metabolism is the most important determinant of how many calories you expend each day. Basal metabolic rate is the calorie burn without any activity. It is the energy required to think, pump blood about the body, heat or cool the body, and perform all other measures of homeostasis. For the average couch potato the basal metabolic rate probably accounts for 80% of the calories burned each day. For professional athletes it accounts for closer to 50%. Joe's problem is that our metabolisms slow down.

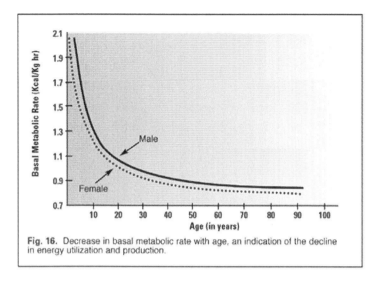

Fig. 16. Decrease in basal metabolic rate with age, an indication of the decline in energy utilization and production.

The chart above demonstrates that men typically have a higher basal metabolic rate than women. This is created in large part by having a greater muscle mass from having higher testosterone levels. Muscle takes much more energy to keep alive than other body tissues even when it is not working. Joe has kept eating the same amount despite having a lower muscle mass and getting older. Either of these factors will cause weight gain.

Recall from chapter three that food is one of the great sources of pleasure in life. The fact that our metabolisms slow with age is thus a depressing aspect of the human condition. We can choose to continue to get the same pleasure from eating in the moment and thus gain weight, which causes decreased pleasure in the future; or, we can choose to invest and have less pleasure in the moment by eating less and be rewarded in the future with the benefits of better health. And better vanity. Of some small secondary benefit, it is less expensive to fuel the body as time goes on as well.

Referring back to the graphic on metabolic change over time, you can see that basal metabolic rate is a moving target. What is working at age 35 will not work at age 40. What is working well at age 60 will not work at age 70. As the metabolic rate is always changing, ever lower, ever lower, the plan of how much food is required to fuel the body must also always be changing, ever lower, ever lower.

Chapter: 7

Medical School

*"Those who are well have no need of a
physician, but those who are sick.
I came not to call the righteous, but sinners."*
Matthew 9:12-13, Mark 2:17, Luke 5:31-32

At the end of college I almost joined the United States Navy. I had gone through the interviews, the physicals, the background checks, and received my commission papers. I was going to join the Navy because my Dad had been a naval officer and the Navy was going to pay my way through medical school. It was a good offer. But, I had a potentially better deal in the works.

The tax-payers of the State of Oregon would occasionally pay the tuition of a student attending Osteopathic Medical School out of state. I applied for just such a scholarship from the State of Oregon. Two days before my Naval commission papers were due the State scholarship came through. As a tradeoff I would have to sacrifice going to my top choice of medical schools. The scholarship only applied to the school near the bottom of my list. I went with the Oregon scholarship (thank you State of Oregon tax payers) and hoped for the best.

Things did not start off very well in medical school. The school was starting a new pilot program where some of the top students would come to the school early and take a two month intensive summer anatomy class and then assist in teaching their own class gross anatomy during the normal academic year. Administration hoped that the normal one-year-long anatomy class could be condensed into two months, but as this had not been tried in the past it was a bit of an experiment. Requirements for entry to the pilot program were a good GPA (which I had), and an "A" in college anatomy. This posed a problem as I had never actually taken anatomy. I had concentrated on classes I could not get in medical school like philosophy, human sexuality, economics, investments, and political science. There were not enough qualified applicants to the program. After being asked to apply based upon my non-anatomy attributes I was subsequently accepted.

I moved to Los Angeles County two months before normal class started, ready to roll up my sleeves and get to work. On introduction day we were given an overview and a tour and then told to return tomorrow with all of the bones memorized. This did not sound too hard. After all, I had broken a lot of bones so I knew the name of some of them. It turns out there are 206 bones in the human body. It also turns out that each bone has nooks and knobs and crevices and turns, and that each of these has a name we were to know as well. I was behind before class ever started.

College had prepared me well for critical thinking and distinguishing the nuances of the various American Premium Lagers. I have never been particularly gifted in memorization. Unfortunately, anatomy is mostly memorization. So, for perhaps the first time in my academic life, I worked hard. What I lacked in rote memorization I more than made up for in the anatomy lab. There was a job to be done of taking a dead person and cutting them up and examining all of the parts. This has to be done in a way that maintains the structures uniquely. All hamburger looks about the same and a heavy handed medical student with a scalpel can make a body into some hamburger pretty fast.

I had been trained by my plastic surgeon Father to clean fish. I have cleaned thousands of fish. In many ways dissecting a human is easier. Human skin is easier to pull away from the underling fat. Human bones are harder to cut through unintentionally. Human organs are larger and thus easier to see. I had the back muscles dissected on day number one faster than some of my smarter but less experienced classmates had learned how to hold a scalpel. And ultimately the class went well, and so did the next, and the next after that. The process of tutoring my classmates in anatomy proved once again that I learn more from teaching than from trying to learn. The founder of my profession, Dr. Andrew Taylor Still, said the three most important things to learn were anatomy, anatomy, and anatomy. Having been pounded into my head, anatomy has served my patients well.

The first two years of medical school are mostly class work. Overall I found this to be easier than college and had a pleasant amount of free time to spend hosting parties, golfing, making overnight all-nighter trips to Las Vegas, and enjoying sports, girls, and beer. This changes in the second half of medical school when you move into the field of clinics and hospitals and actually start working on rotations. The hours were longer, the pressure higher, and the reward much greater. I loved it.

I chose to travel the country for my rotations. I flew or drove to a new hospital each month. I heard the best ER experience was in the Bronx, so I spent four weeks sleeping on a stained mattress lying on a stained carpet in a very high-crime neighborhood. The roaches mostly ran away if you turned on the lights before you looked. The rats ran away if you walked with a heavy stride. There were drug deals on the corner outside my housing. I saw guns and knives pulled as I walked to work. While not a place I wanted to live, the training was fantastic.

The hospital was severely understaffed. Most of the patients did not have the ability to pay for their care so the hospital did not have the ability to pay for nurses, technicians, secretaries, etc. All of that work was done by the residents, interns, and students. If you wanted blood drawn you did it yourself. Twenty-five percent of the patients were HIV+ and a very high percentage were IV drug users. This makes drawing blood harder as the good veins had been destroyed. So, I would try and try and try again. I would usually give up after six times sticking the patient with a needle, but sooner if they were particularly nice or scary. Then a resident would help, and I would watch and learn. We used scalp veins, neck veins, deep veins, and sometimes just pushed large gauge needles through the scar tissue on the front of the elbow. Smaller needles would bend, but a big thick needle would get through.

My first patient was a cop who had been stabbed in the abdomen after a drug deal he was doing for some extra pocket cash went sour. The resident took a quick peek and then told me to sew him up. I had sewn dead pig's feet in class but I had never sewn a person before. The cop asked my why my hands were shaking. "Too much coffee" I replied. And though my hands shook and my forehead sweated I got the job done without needing any help.

The Bronx was where I delivered by first baby. While working on something else in the back corner of the ER, someone started screaming for help. I thought to myself that someone should really go see what that person needs. I looked up from my less urgent case and saw there were no doctors or nurses around. I investigated myself.

A 26 year-old woman who had lived a very hard life and looked closer to 40 said, "It's coming!" I said "what is coming?" She said "The baby!" I had no idea how to deliver a baby. I started screaming for help too. None came. So, I put on some gloves and acted calm. I used a soothing tone. I said, "It is OK, I am here for you." I sure as hell did not say "push." I did not want that baby to come out while I was in charge. But, the mom was pushing anyway. Eventually she pushed the baby out. One of the residents had quietly shown up over my shoulder and told me not to drop anything. She then instructed me to tie and cut the cord, and then to deliver the placenta. And at the end of this miracle I was certain of something: I never wanted to deliver another baby again.

As I progressed on my journey through school I noted that as the level of academics rises, the rates of agnosticism and atheism increase and the rates of faith decrease. High school teachers are likely to have faith. Doctors are much less likely. Doctors at teaching hospitals are less likely yet. So, as I entered medical school and subsequently the hospitals, I was surrounded by more really smart people who did not believe in God and fewer people who went to church. My search for greater meaning to life slowed and my investment in better understanding how this life functions increased. Even then I found it interesting that we studied how to keep the body alive longer, but there was no teaching about the obvious fact that all bodies will perish.

That conversation has come more from a political and social arena with programs such as "death with dignity," the "Oregon suicide law," and the President's "death panels." The goal of all of these programs is to admit that death will happen, and then have a conversation about how to make it happen as best fits the wishes of the dying person. People don't like to talk about death. They do not like reminders of mortality. It causes fear and raises hard questions about life. But I like hard questions.

On a rotation in Texas, I met Stacey as we both trained in the same hospital in Corpus Christi. She was a God-fearing Texas girl. Her faith was clearly of paramount importance to her and she communicated very clearly that she was willing to die for her faith. I asked her why she believed in God. She replied, essentially "Because my parents said to." I asked her questions about her faith and she would only use the Bible to give evidence. I asked her why the Bible should be a source of authority and her answer was, "Because the Bible says so." She did not seem keen to explore the idea of a circular argument. I gave her the example of me saying that she should listen to me because God is speaking to her through me, and to prove it, it is because I say it is so. Stacey was not impressed.

I asked her about the miracles in the Bible: the parting of the Red Sea, Jesus walking on water, and people rising from death. Wasn't it more likely that these stories are creations of man? She had no answer. I asked about the sinless Buddhist monk. How could a God worth serving condemn that harmless meditating man to hell? I asked about her view on creation. She took a hard line biblical view that the world was not very old. She did not have a good explanation of the dinosaurs. She did not have a refutation for carbon dating or for evolutionary theory. She did not know about Aristotle's answer to creation. She could not refute or co-opt big bang theory. In fact, it seemed as if this highly intelligent doctor-in-training, the one who had to take all the same science classes I had taken for medical school prep, had never even thought about the questions I asked her.

I also asked questions about the actions of the faithful and the church. I asked about the Anabaptist killings, the crusades, use of God to justify war, bombings of abortion clinics, pedophile priests, and Jim Bakker and the thousand others like him. Did the abominable actions of the faithful reflect on the faith?

I also asked about scripture itself. Why is the last supper on a different day in the Gospel of John than in the other three books? Why does the Gospel of Matthew have Judas hang himself and the priests buy the potter's field while, inconsistently, Luke, in the book of Acts, has Judas buy the field and then his guts burst forth? Why is the order of creation different in Genesis 1 and Genesis 2? Why is scripture polytheistic until the last book of the Pentateuch? If the Bible is the inspired word of God then it seems like there should be no inconsistencies.

Ultimately our "discussion" ended in tears. To this day I am not sure if this is because I asked questions that made her question her own faith, or more likely that she mourned for my soul. I was hoping that Stacey would be able to help me wrestle with some hard questions. But, truthfully, the scoffing part of me enjoyed trying to make her wrestle, too. She honestly tried to help and I made her cry.

This was one of many "discussions" with Christians that filled me with more doubt than faith. Why could they be so sure of something seemingly without ever having thought about it? It was not just lay-people that left me with this feeling. Priests and pastors were not much more compelling. Their argument always started one of two places. Option "A" was to look to scripture. But that was not a path I was very willing to walk down until scripture itself had been proven as a reliable source of something. Follow-up arguments for this were weak. Option "B" was to say faith is given through grace by God. I thus just needed to have faith and trust in God. This was not helpful either. I had hard questions to deal with in regards to God. The idea that these hard questions would best be dealt with by me trying harder to have faith left me feeling both inadequate and more skeptical.

Chapter: 8

Science Lesson #4 –
Diet Pills and Shots

"Food gained by fraud tastes sweet, but one ends up with a mouth full of gravel." Proverbs 20:17

In my quest to avoid my fate of fatness I have looked into every medication possible to see if there may be a gem. There have been a lot of diets, diet pills, and diet shots over the centuries. Some, like taking excessive thyroid hormone, have seemed like an intuitively bad idea from the start. Others, like a THC (marijuana) receptor blocker, have seemed promising. Yet others, like injecting placental hormone, have seemed bizarre. I am just fine with bizarre as long as it is effective.

Jenifer came to see me having been overweight her entire life. Well, almost. She was born a few weeks early and had trouble gaining weight as a very young infant. The doctors taught her parents that it was very important for her to eat enough calories for

41

her to be able to thrive. Her loving parents performed as ordered and fed her and fed her. Even though Jenifer was doing fine by two months of age her parents never really switched off the goal of feeding her enough. By age six months she was overweight. She has been that way ever since.

Jenifer has tried a few diets. They led to weight loss every time. They also led to weight gain every time she stopped the diet. Jenifer now wants to try the HCG diet. It worked great for a friend of hers who lost 40 pounds. HCG stands for human chorionic gonadotropin and there are currently 10,000 HCG weight loss clinics in the USA. It is the hormone made by the placenta of pregnant women which turns a pregnancy test positive. The HCG diet combines severe calorie restriction (500 calories a day) along with HCG shots and reliably leads to weight loss in both men and women.

It may seem odd to inject a placenta hormone as a means of weight loss. The diet claims to raise testosterone levels through the HCG shots. The diet claims to curb hunger. The diet claims to speed up the metabolism. The diet claims that you will lose fat and not muscle. The problem with these claims is that they are not true. For women, this diet has been studied in placebo-controlled blinded trials where neither the researchers nor the participants knew who was getting the real HCG and who was getting the placebo HCG. There was no benefit to weight loss. No benefit to hunger is demonstrable. No benefit to metabolic rate was seen. Both the placebo and the HCG arms of the study lost the same amount of weight.

For the HCG to work there has to be testicles. As females lack testicles, there is no effect of raising testosterone levels from HCG for women. The claims of the diet are thus false. But, why then are there 10,000 HCG clinics across the United States? It is because they are selling hope, and hope is a very valuable commodity. It is also because the diet works. The HCG diet consists of eating 500 calories a day in addition to the hormone shot. An intake of 500 calories is much less than the body burns in a day. The mismatch between the intake and the output leads to weight loss. It just does not lead to any more weight loss than the same diet without the hormone shot.

The HCG wasn't the first popular low calorie diet. In the 1970's The Cambridge Diet was very popular and consistently successful in leading to weight loss. The diet called for reducing caloric intake to 320 calories per day. The Cambridge Diet led to significant weight loss for as long as people were on the diet. The problem is that people died while on this diet. The Food and Drug Administration (FDA) shut the Cambridge Diet down after 58 deaths. The total protein intake on this low calorie intake is too low to support life. Participants literally starved to death.

Speaking of deadly diets, there have been quite a few. During World War I, observers noted that fat men who worked in the munitions plants and came in contact with a chemical called dinitrophenol lost significant weight. Russia used the drug in WWI to keep cold soldiers warm. It helps with this process by increasing metabolic rate. The main side effect seen in the Russian soldiers was weight loss. By 1935 over 100,000 Americans had taken dinitrophenol as a weight loss drug. It was advertised as a "new and safe" way to lose weight. It was removed by the FDA in 1938 due to its significant ill effects including death. The drug served as example in the "chamber of horrors" exhibit that led to the Food, Drug, and Cosmetic Act of 1938. It epitomizes an example of a weight loss drug that burns the candle much brighter, which leads to both weight loss and also unfavorable side effects like seizures, arrhythmias, and death.

Dinitrophenol made a comeback in the 1980s in Texas. It was sold in Physicians Clinics under the name Mictal by Dr. Nicholas Bachynsky. He was Russian-born and worked for the US federal government for some time translating Russian documents. He learned of the weight loss properties of dinitrophenol when he was carrying out these translations. These weight loss clinics were big business for Dr. Bachynsky. Fourteen-thousand patrons were paying up to $1300 per month for his weight loss remedy. His patients all signed consent forms for use of the dinitrophenol despite the known risks of cataract formation, fever, blood clots, and death. These risks were known because of all of the cases of such problems with use of the drug in the 1930's. Some patients died of body temperatures increasing to 110 degrees Fahrenheit (43.3 Celsius), many developed blindness at very young ages from aggressive cataract formation. The State of Texas eventually shut down Dr. Bachynsky's business three years after complaints of side effects of the Mictal first rang into the local poison control centers.

Kellogg's Safe Fat Reducer is another example of a weight loss remedy that burns the metabolic candle brighter. In 1910, this remedy was marketed by the cereal company as a safe means of weight loss. Mr. Kellogg would send the first box of his $1 Safe Fat Reducer for free. He claimed that it would reduce fat "without tiresome exercise", and do it "safely" while aiding in digestion. It contained thyroxine, more commonly known as thyroid hormone, and a laxative. Taking too much thyroid hormone does lead to weight loss. Unfortunately it also leads to potentially fatal irregular heartbeats, strokes, inability to sleep, osteoporosis, diarrhea, and tremors. This diet was heavily advertised in newspapers and was taken by tens of thousands of hopeful customers. The federal government insisted on the removal of the thyroid hormone due to safety concerns, but the diet continued to be sold for years by Kellogg's, containing nothing more than laxatives and bread crumbs.

Still looking at early 20th century weight loss remedies, Dexedrine is another example of an agent that works by burning the metabolic candle brighter. Dexedrine is the D (right-handed) isomer of amphetamine. It began to be used for weight loss in the 1930s. To know the side effects of taking amphetamine it is useful to look at the effect of methamphetamine on meth users. Rapid heart rate, dilated pupils, aggressiveness, irritability, hallucinations, skin picking, elevation of blood pressure, elevation of body temperature, diarrhea, twitching, heart attack, stroke, convulsions, and death are all possibilities. Dexedrine was marketed heavily in the 1960s and 1970s as a safe means of weight loss. It was removed from the market due to safety concerns after numerous adverse outcomes. Dexedrine was subsequently remarketed as a treatment for attention deficit disorder in the 1990s and remains FDA-approved for that purpose at present time.

Together, all of the examples of weight loss remedies which cause a temporary increase in metabolic activity as their mechanism of action present a pattern. All of that class of medication has proven to be either unsafe or ineffective. Often both. In general, the stimulant class of weight loss pills falls into the effective but unsafe category. Fen-phen is an example. The drug was marketed for weight loss and also tested for helping with cocaine and alcohol addiction. It was shown to be effective for both in rats. For humans it does work for weight loss in most people through suppression of appetite and a revving of the metabolism. The phen (phentermine) portion of the Fen-phen has side effects similar to the amphetamines and the other stimulants previously discussed. The fen (fenfluramine) portion worked uniquely to the previously discussed agents in that it increased serotonin levels. This leads to less hunger and thus weight loss.

Unfortunately, fen-phen also has a unique side effect of causing elevated blood pressure on the lungs and problems with heart valves. There was controversy at the FDA even before the drug was approved. It was already being used in Europe for weight loss and had been shown prior to FDA approval to be associated with increased risk of raising blood pressure in the lungs leading to an incurable condition called pulmonary hypertension which causes shortness of breath and ultimately death. Despite this, the FDA approved the drug and within three months there were almost 100,000 prescriptions a week being written in the US, and there were 18,000,000 patients, including my grandmother, taking the drug by 1996.

In 1997, the Mayo Clinic and *The New England Journal of Medicine* released data showing that fen-phen was associated with an increased risk of heart valve problems. A follow-up study showed that an astonishing 30% of fen-phen users had abnormal echocardiograms (heart ultrasounds) and fen-phen was pulled from the market. Since that time an estimated $12,000,000,000 has been paid out in claims related to harm caused from fen-phen side effects.

One month after fen-phen was pulled from the market Meridia, was introduced. Structurally similar to amphetamines, Meridia increases levels of pleasure neurotransmitters in the brain and thus curbs hunger. Meridia is less effective as a weight loss agent than more potent stimulants and it was thought to perhaps be safer. It was pulled from the market in most countries after a study on safety showed a high risk of heart attack and strokes. Seizures and diarrhea, high blood pressure and numbness, arrhythmia and paralysis are all known side effects as well.

In my adult lifetime the first drug that appeared promising for weight loss was a THC receptor blocker. THC is the active drug in marijuana. Consuming marijuana gave my fellow college students the munchies. The idea of blocking that receptor therefore seemed intuitively appealing to me. In addition, this was a novel idea. All of the other weight loss agents were either stimulants (dangerous and effective or dangerous and ineffective depending on the agent), laxatives (lose water weight only and in a messy fashion), or a waste of money and effort (placebo). At least this was something new. My concern when I first read about the idea was the other effects of blocking that receptor. There is a reason people chose to smoke marijuana, and it is not for weight gain. Blocking that pleasure receptor seemed to have the intrinsic risk of decreasing pleasure. It is a risk that someone like me may be willing to bear however, if the pleasure gained from maintaining an ideal weight would be greater than the displeasure of the drug.

Acomplia, a CB1 THC receptor blocker, was released in Europe in 2006 after showing favorable results in studies for weight loss. The drug manufacturer submitted application for approval through the FDA for release in the US, but was denied due to lack of proof of safety of the agent. The drug was removed from the market in 2008 after it was found to cause mental disorders including severe depression, psychosis, and suicide.

I am not a lover of history. But, I think the idea of taking a pill or shot or potion with the goal of weight loss should be viewed through the lens of history. There have been thousands of weight loss remedies marketed in the past 100 years. All of them have been a bad idea. All of them. If there were a single counterexample then the epidemic of obesity would not be an epidemic. If there were a single safe and effective pill or potion then everyone would know about it. The fact there has never been such a drug despite the investment of hundreds of billions of dollars and thousands of failures suggests that there never will be a safe and effective drug for weight loss. There are things that do work for weight loss. There are appropriate targets of our hope. These would be a better option on which to place your faith.

Chapter: 9

The Jesus Problem

"The fear of the LORD is the beginning of wisdom, And the knowledge of the Holy One is understanding." Proverbs 9:10

As I was learning to drive there were not many days available to get practice driving in the snow. In Portland, Oregon it snows very rarely. Some years it does not snow at all. Both of my parents are from Minnesota where there is snow on the ground for most of the winter and often most of the spring as well. To them, it was an important part of learning to drive that I should know how to drive in the snow and ice. The opportunity came while we were on a family vacation in the mountains. I got the chance to drive back to the cabin from a dinner at the lodge.

I drove pretty well until I hit an ice patch. Everyone in the car could feel the loss of traction. This caused my soprano Mother to begin to scream at the top of her lungs from the back seat. It caused my Father to reach across and grab the steering wheel. Neither of these helpful actions by my parents saved the day. We crashed into a tree. I am still glad the tree was there because three feet to the right or left we would have slid off the road down a steep embankment.

I sat embarrassed with wounded pride. Wounded pride often leads to sinful behavior. You may know someone who has a defense mechanism of going on the attack. "The best defense is a good offense." A mistake of some sort will happen and as a result a person with this mentality will launch into one of a couple of options. One possibility is a string of reasons why it is not their fault. It was the "ice on the road," or "these antilock brakes don't allow you to skid like the old brakes did," or "there was some glare from the snow." There is a deeper level of lack of responsibility here as well which may sound something like "if you had not been screaming, touching the wheel, or making me angry, then I would not have made a mistake." It takes the finger off of the individual and the circumstances and points it at someone else. Notice how none of these sounds like "I am sorry I was driving faster than I should have been and crashed."

After nine years into my search for the meaning of life and the chief end of man I had gained the ability to argue why things may not be true. I could ask really hard questions such as, "Why is man made in 'our' image in Genesis Chapter One? Who is this 'our'?" How does the believer reconcile the polytheistic Enuma Elis, the oldest recorded creation story, with Genesis? Why not until chapter four of the last book of the Pentateuch do we see the first glimpse of monotheism in the Bible? The Ten Commandments says to "put no other gods before me?" This implies that there are other gods. Why does it not just say, "Hey stupid, there are no other gods, so quit offending me and wasting your time by offering sacrifice to them?"

Reading apologetics such as "*The Will to Believe*" by William James where it is argued that I/we should believe because it would be good for me/us to do so were not persuasive. I did not want to believe something unless it was true, and I would want to believe in a true something even if it were harmful for me to do so. I was a bit stuck. So, God sent me something that had the ability to get through to my heart. God sent girls.

I had come to most 'conversations' about faith and religion with fighting gloves on. When lips and breasts were involved I was put in a place where I was listening differently. Katie brought up the question of my faith early in our relationship. She was quite interested to learn that I was an agnostic, deistic, hedonistic, confirmed Catholic. We went through each of those terms and I explained how each fit. When I asked hard questions about reconciling the creation story and evolutionary theory she was fit to answer in a way that kept my BS meter from ringing. When I asked questions about the sins of the church and Christians in general she pointed out that Christians remain sinful and the church, being a collection of sinful Christians, should not be expected to be any different.

When I asked how her scientific mind could reconcile Hume's treatise *Of Miracles* with the miracles in scripture she said she would get back to me. This time I was handed a copy of *Mere Christianity* by C.S. Lewis. Recall the start of this journey when I was concussed by the revelation that I was fated to be obese. Lewis rocked me similarly. By this time I had spent 10 years asking people about the meaning of life and I remain a bit angry that through all of the meetings, discussions, reading, and arguing that nobody had presented me with what I now call The Jesus Problem.

Who was Jesus? Was he a prophet, a nice guy, a religious leader, kind to children, and probably a good fisherman? Was he, in essence, a good guy, but not necessarily divine? Lewis pointed out this is not a logically tenable position. Jesus claims to be the Son of God (see the gospels of Matthew, Luke, and especially John). You cannot reasonably deny the deity of Jesus without reading the gospel accounts first. Jesus claims he will rise from the dead to judge the living and the dead. These are not the claims of a "good guy." These are not claims that a "good religious leader" gets to make. Lewis argued very well that Jesus has to be "lunatic" or "Lord."

If a friend were to say to you "I am the Son of God and I am going to rise from the dead in three days and be seated at the right hand of my Father (God) and later return to judge you!" you would think they had gone off of the deep end. Insanity (lunatic) would be a logical position to hold with regard to Jesus as well. Lewis postulates that the other viable logical option is that Jesus is exactly who he says he was. Jesus is Lord. He is the Son of God, who was given by God to be killed on the cross for the forgiveness of our broken relationship with God, and who will come again to judge the living and the dead.

Lewis had me. I again felt knocked upside the head. How had I gotten one of the rare A's in my class on predicate and quantifier logic and not seen this myself? How had I been meeting with priests and pastors and reading apologetics and asking hard questions of Christians for years and not come across this before? It made me feel a bit better to know that someone with the genius of Lewis, who had been a devout atheist, had not wrestled with this question himself until about age 30, subsequently converting heart and soul to Christianity. As I looked over his argument I saw a possible flaw. Perhaps Jesus never existed and/or he was just a construct of the church.

I asked for evidence about authenticity of scripture. Katie admitted that it was a very good question for which she did not have an answer but that she would look into it. She came back with the Dead Sea Scrolls, Suetonius and *The Twelve Caesars* written in 112AD, Tacitus and *The Annals of Imperial Rome* written in 116AD, Thallus' commentary on the crucifixion and his errant explanation of an eclipse in 52AD, and Josephus' *Antiquities of the Jews*, written 94AD. Individually each provided evidence for historical authenticity of scripture. Taken as a group the evidence seemed compelling.

Thallus provided my favorite writing of the bunch. He attempted to debunk the darkness that took place at the time of the crucifixion by suggesting a total eclipse of the sun. This idea was quickly shown to be impossible due to the full moon at the time of Passover. The moon and the sun have to be diametrically opposed for a full moon, thus making it impossible for them to be diametrically aligned to create an eclipse. Note the lunar position for a full moon and a solar eclipse:

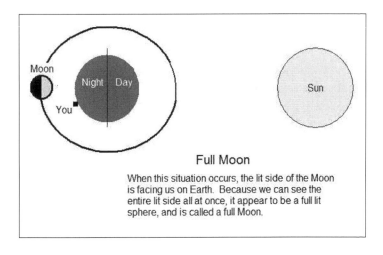

Full Moon

When this situation occurs, the lit side of the Moon is facing us on Earth. Because we can see the entire lit side all at once, it appear to be a full lit sphere, and is called a full Moon.

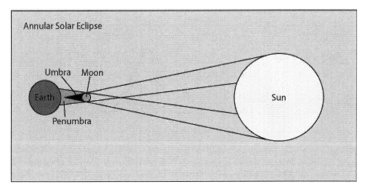

By errantly attempting to give a natural explanation for the darkness having been caused by an eclipse, Thallus inadvertently accomplished a couple of things. First, he established that Jesus was a real man that lived and was crucified. Second, it became dark at the time of the crucifixion, in fact dark enough to be a total eclipse of the sun. That type of darkness would be miraculous. Thallus thus gives credibility to both Jesus and miracles. While the writings of the apostle Paul do the same thing, Paul does so with a clear bias. Biased people are less believable. This bias is removed in the case of Thallus, which makes his writing on the existence of Jesus more believable.

It did not occur to me at the time, but it is obvious now that the best evidence for the existence of a living Christ is the ongoing effect He is having on the lives of people in the present. It is possible to have a fascination with Karl Marx, Mother Theresa, Adam Smith, Immanuel Kant, Thomas Jefferson, Socrates, Charles Darwin, or Steve Jobs. They will never have the effect on people that Jesus has. They are remembered because of their ideas. Jesus, risen from the dead and still alive, has ongoing divine relationships with people in a way that no dead person can. Jesus changes lives and causes people to be born into a new creation. Even if I did not believe fully myself, I could still see strong evidence of this in others. Even if its effect is off-putting, the power of the gospel to change lives in an active way is simply undeniable.

I now had to solve The Jesus Problem. If he is Lord then I should give all of my life over to Him. If he is liar or lunatic then I should give none of my life over to him. I had reached a true branch point in my journey. Walking down one path would mean walking straight toward Jesus and the cross. It would mean walking toward Jesus seated at the right hand of the father with white hair, feet of bronze, and a giant sword coming out of his mouth. Walking down the other path would mean trying to live the rest of my short life attempting to maximize pleasure and minimize pain. It would also mean pitying the billions of Christians believing in a lie. Pascal's Wager had never struck me as a very good argument as at the root it seemed all self-serving. Pascal's idea is that if God is real and you obey him you are in good shape. If you do not, you are going to hell. If God is not real and you obey him you are still in OK shape. If God is not real and you do not obey him then you gambled and won. The wager of not following God is not a good one to make as there is little to gain and a life in hell to lose. I was now looking at a God-serving version of Pascal's Wager. Then along came another girl.

Chapter: 10

Science Lesson #5 – Medical Causes of a Slow Metabolism Exist – Make Sure You Don't Have One

"Do you not know that your bodies are temples of the Holy Spirit, who is in you, whom you have received from God? You are not your own; you were bought at a price. Therefore honor God with your bodies." 1 Corinthians 6:19-20

Part way through my sports medicine fellowship I worked with a surgeon clearly frustrated by what he perceived to be a lack of self-responsibility in overweight patients. If patients expressed any resistance to his suggestion of weight loss he would go into his Auschwitz diatribe:

"Do you see any fat people in the concentration camps? Show me just one person coming out of the concentration

> camps that was fat and then we can keep talking about
> how you can't lose weight. I mean if people who eat 'basi-
> cally nothing' like you do stay fat, why were there not a
> bunch of fat people in the concentration camps?"

I am still a bit shocked that he would say such a thing. It came across like a slap to the patient's face...exactly how it was intended. His point was very well taken by me. It is common for patients to say things like "I hardly eat anything," or "I eat almost nothing" while weighing twice what would be good for them. Such statements are hard to believe, so hard in fact that it may provoke anger in the person hearing such a statement. So I appreciate the Auschwitz example as proof that if you really don't eat much, then it seems unlikely that you would still be gaining weight.

However, it is true that some people eat quite a bit more food than others to keep themselves alive. What creates this difference? Does "I hardly eat anything" really mean "I eat a lot less than I see other people eating and it seems unfair?" There are two basic components involved here. The first and most important is the metabolism (see chapter five) which determines the vast majority of energy usage for most adults. The other component is activity. This is not just exercise but any activity. Even thinking requires energy and thus burns calories.

As the metabolism is the major determinant of calorie usage it makes sense to get it checked out and to ensure that it is optimized. There are a number of factors that can slow it down and I know a few tricks to get it humming along a bit faster. First though, some data will be needed.

I like data. Data leaves feelings out of the equation. "Do you think I'm fat?" is a matter of opinion. Cholesterol = 229 is a statement of fact. Body fat = 31% is a statement of fact. Here are the facts I recommend collecting:

Lipid Profile (cholesterol panel) – this is a measure of underlying metabolic health and is a known risk factor for heart attacks, strokes, and many other forms of blood vessel problems.

Blood Sugar – this is the main fuel of the body. Having too little around is fatal. Having too much is diabetes which is also fatal, but on a slower time scale.

Body Fat Percentage – this is a much more accurate measure of fatness than a scale or measuring tape or BMI (body mass index). There are a variety of ways to measure this such as caliper tests, underwater weight, impedance, DEXA, CT scan, the egg, and MRI scan. All are reasonably accurate. During my fellowship we did the majority of these tests on each other and all were within 1% error for me.

Body Mass Index – a measure of weight relative to height. It can be misleading for individuals with lots of muscle mass, but it is a good measure for the non-athlete.

Resting Heart Rate – a cheap and easy measure of cardiovascular fitness. The lower the number of heart beats per minute the better the fitness.

Blood Pressure – a measure of the pressure in the pipes. Again, too low is fatal. Too high is hypertension which is another well-known risk factor for blood vessel problems such as heart attack and stroke.

In addition to the above items if you are struggling with your weight it would be prudent to get your metabolic rate checked. There are a number of components to a metabolism. The most important is the basal metabolic rate. This is the rate you burn calories when you are doing nothing such as lying in bed at rest. This can be checked at a human performance lab and costs around $100. It varies significantly from person to person. If a human performance lab is not available then there are some ways to fudge an answer:

Basal Metabolic Rate Based Upon Weight -

Men: BMR = 66 + (13.7 * wt in kg) + (5 * ht in cm) - (6.8 * age in years)

Women: BMR = 655 + (9.6 * wt in kg) + (1.8 * ht in cm) - (4.7 * age in years)

1 inch = 2.54 cm.

1 kilogram = 2.2 lbs.

Example: 30 year old female, 5'6" (167.6cm), 120lb (54.5 kilos)

BMR = 655 + 523 + 302 - 141 = **1339 calories/day**

BMR based on lean body weight (if body fat percentage is known, this is a more accurate equation):

Men and Women: BMR = 370 + (21.6 * lean mass in kg)
Example: 30 year old female, 5'6" (167.6cm), 120lb (54.5 kilos)
Your BMR = 370 + (21.6 * 43.6) = **1312 calories**

Variables that control the basal metabolic rate can be checked as well. Ask your doctor to consider the following:

Thyroid Function – this is a measure of the hormone that controls all aspects of metabolism for the entire body. Thyroid disorders are relatively common. An under-functioning thyroid is a common cause of weight gain.

Vitamin D – the sunshine vitamin. There is a vitamin D receptor on every cell in the body and its presence is necessary for normal metabolic function. Vitamin D deficiency causes slowing of the basal metabolism.

Two Hour Glucose Tolerance Test – this is a measure of how well your body metabolizes carbohydrates. After not eating for many hours the blood sugar is checked in the fasting state, then 75 grams of glucose is consumed (about the same as 20oz of soda), then the blood sugar is rechecked in two hours. A normal carbohydrate metabolism will show the blood sugar to be normal under fasting conditions and normal two hours after consuming the glucose. If either blood sugar is high it is a sign of poor carbohydrate metabolism and perhaps diabetes. It is very hard to lose weight if the blood sugar is high.

Fasting and Two Hour Insulin Level – this is a measure of how much insulin the body has to make in order to keep the blood sugar regulated. Insulin is made in the pancreas and it is a growth factor. More insulin = more fat, hair, skin tags, and sometimes skin pigment (dark colored skin around the neck, arm pits, and other skin folds called acanthosis nigricans). It is another measure of carbohydrate metabolism and is often abnormal long before the blood sugar itself becomes abnormal. It is very difficult to lose weight if the insulin level is high.

Cortisol – this is produced by glands just above the kidneys call the adrenals. Too much cortisol leads to high blood pressure and weight gain. The weight gained from cortisol excess tends to be present centrally in the belly and back and face.

Core Body Temperature – this is a measure of how hot the furnace runs. It is a very inexpensive measure of a component of basal metabolic rate. Metabolic rate increases by about 5% for each degree Fahrenheit of body temperature increase. This is why the dinitrophenol discussed in chapter four works for weight loss. It also helps to explain why well-insulated people would feel colder in a given room than thin people when it may otherwise be assumed that all of that insulation would cause one to be unbearably hot. Whales and walruses are able to swim around in cold water due to the insulating properties of blubber. If you are overweight and cold, the problem is not a lack of insulation.

Sleep study – this is a measure of sleep quality. It is performed at home or in a sleep lab. About one-third of life is spent asleep and sleep quality and quantity are both important to metabolic health. Sleep apnea is present in around ten percent of adult men and five percent of adult women. Kids can have it as well. Sleep apnea is having pauses in breathing while sleeping. It is very damaging to the metabolism. Fifty percent of people with high blood pressure have sleep apnea. If you are trying hard to lose weight and it is not working, consider talking to your doctor about a sleep study.

Waist Circumference – this is how big around you are one inch above the belly button. 40 inches and over for men and 35 inches and over for women is considered obesity. This is a better measure of metabolic health than a BMI (body mass index) as it takes into consideration where the weight is carried. Weight carried in the midsection is more likely to be harmful than weight carried in the arms and legs.

When I check the metabolism of overweight patients in my office the majority have an identifiable flaw. Your doctor may recommend other measures of metabolic health as well and wonderful new tests may be just around the corner and available as measures of more data soon. All of these measures of metabolic health are a tool to gauge the body. Empower yourself with some data and you will have at your disposal a powerful tool for affecting change.

Chapter: 11

Trying on Jesus to See How He Fits

"The fear of the Lord is the beginning of wisdom" Proverbs 111:10

There are a variety of ways to help make hard decisions. Lists of advantages and disadvantages can help. Seeking the opinion of people you respect can help. Sleeping on it can help. If possible, gathering more information is a good idea as well. Taking a car for a test drive is an example of this. If you can't decide between the minivan and the station wagon, drive each of them to see which you prefer. If both wedding dresses look equally good on the hanger, then try them on and see how they twirl as you dance.

Well, I had a very big decision to make. Was Jesus God? Or, was Jesus a fraud? I did not want to choose based upon which suited me better as I twirled. I wanted to choose truth. There were plenty of really smart and compelling people on both sides of this issue so seeking the opinion of others sounded exhausting and unhelpful at the same time. I was still a bit upset with myself for existing for years in a foolish position of having a partial belief in Jesus when it really needed to be an all or nothing affair. I did not want to languish in a state of indecision. I wanted to find the true path and walk it.

My pro-con list included the ramifications of choosing errantly. If I walked the path of rejecting Jesus first and it was the wrong path then I would be making a potentially grave mistake. If I walked the path of faith and found it to be false then I could simply jump to the other path of absolute hedonism with little implication. To the outside observer I am not sure that my behavior would look that much different. On the path of hedonism I would be choosing based upon what brought me the most pleasure. Well, I like doing things that are nice for other people. I like being honest. I like honoring my mother and father. I like going to class and getting good grades. Speeding and drugs and promiscuous sex make me uncomfortable and thus hold little or no appeal to me. While my behavior would not look much different, the motivation behind the behavior would be antithetical. The path of Jesus would mean loss of control, the path of apostasy would mean absolute control. Then along came another girl.

I imagine God muttering to himself "my goodness that Karl is stubborn...I will have to place something before him that he cannot resist." I had dated girls that were nice and pretty and smart and sexy and funny before. But never like this one. Her name was Amy and she uniquely stirred a desire in me to be a better man. Amy stood firmly on only one path, the path of faith. She held out her hand to me and asked me to follow her. My decision had become easy. The path itself however was not as efficient to travel as I would have liked.

The nature of faith is interesting. Everyone believes in something. Some people believe in a political party. If only everyone thought like they do, then, so they believe, everything would be better. Some people believe in education. If only everyone were more aware and educated to a higher level, then mankind would be able to climb above war and poverty. Others believe in science. Through technology and scientific advancement we will be able to move society forward. Others believe in absence of a god. Ashes to ashes and dust to dust. Absolute proof for any of these beliefs is lacking. So what is belief? What is faith?

The apostle Paul points out that "hope that is seen is not hope. For who hopes for what he sees (Romans 8:24)?" Hope points to faith as something that cannot be seen or known with certainty. Certainty implies a complete or absolute knowledge, which is exactly what is not found in something requiring faith. The author of Hebrews states, "Now faith is the assurance of things hoped for, the conviction of things not seen (Hebrews 11:1)." I was seeking to have faith, to believe in Jesus as Son of God and Son of Man, but I did not know how to make that happen. All of my reasons for doubt had not simply disappeared. Amy was there to help.

Her suggestion was to live as if I believed fully. Take every risk. Jump in with both feet. She gave me a somewhat useful picture of a man standing on solid footing at the edge of a deep and dark chasm. The other side of the chasm could not be clearly seen. There was some evidence that it was there, but not certainty. Faith she said "is like jumping with hope and trust across that chasm." It will be uncomfortable. It will feel risky. It will require doubts to be laid aside.

So I jumped. I prayed for forgiveness of my sins and my doubts. I prayed to accept Jesus as my Lord and Savior. And..........I really did not feel much different. I went to church every Sunday, read the Bible, prayed, and tried to behave as if I believed fully. And still............I did not feel much different. I went to altar calls for people turning their lives to Jesus and I raised my hand when the pastor asked to be able to pray for those hoping to turn their lives to Jesus. And still.........I did not feel much different. Oh, my measure of faith grew a bit; it just was not a conversion experience. Some people simply have to hear the good news of Jesus and they say, "Oh my, that is wonderful!" They are born again, and in one moment they are changed. For me it was more like an ultra-marathon.

Years passed while on this march. I took Amy off of the free market by marrying her as fast as I could convince her. I finished my residency. I finished my sports medicine fellowship. We started having babies. And still I marched, with Amy encouraging and holding my hand and my heart every step of the way. While marching on this path my measure of doubt very slowly decreased and my measure of faith increased. And then God answered a prayer.

Chapter: 12

Science Lesson #6 – Fourth Grade Math and Department Store Mirrors

*"When they measure themselves by themselves
and compare themselves with themselves,
they are not wise."* 2 Corinthians 10:12

I play in a weekly Saturday 6:30am basketball game. I love it for it's good sportsmanship that is not devoid of competition. My friend Lawrence wears a strap around his chest which communicates with his wristwatch. It very accurately measures his heart rate. It also has a calorie counting mechanism. It is always a topic of conversation at the end of the game "Hey Larry! How many did we burn today?" Over the course of two hours of vigorous basketball the watch will say that Larry has burned as many as 2000 calories. Some exercise equipment at the gym has similar calorie counting systems. I have been quite pleased to burn 300 calories on the elliptical machine in a mere 8 minutes. These watches and exercise machines are like department store mirrors.

Remember the mirrors in fun houses at the amusement park or the fair? They can make you fat, short, tall, or thin. Some of them do a little of all of this at different parts. At the department store when you are trying on your dress to see if it looks good it is common to look in the mirror. The store knows this. They will put in mirrors that are just a little bit slimming. Not fun house slimming, but just enough to help convince you that the dress looks good enough to buy. The exercise equipment is using a similar trick. By telling you that you are burning gobs of calories, you like the product better. You are thus more inclined to use it, buy it, and recommend it. It is great for business but may not be good for the waistline.

It is time to brush up your fourth grade math skills. Addition, subtraction, and simple multiplication are involved. Some of the variables will make you uncomfortable. And that is exactly the intent.

Burning Calories:
- 1 mile run = 100 calories
- 1 mile walked = 100 calories
- 1 mile jogged = 100 calories

It does not matter how you do it, moving yourself one mile on your own feet burns about 100 calories. I get some funny looks from patients when discussing this. Having done both, they are pretty sure that running is harder than walking. How then could walking burn the same number of calories as running? Well, it just takes longer. A fast runner like my wife may run a mile in 6 minutes. A jogger will run a mile in 12 minutes. A walker will walk a mile in 18 minutes. Based upon units of time the runner will burn three times as many calories as the walker and that is why running feels harder. It is harder. But each group will still burn the same calories per mile traveled.

This is very helpful. Calorie burn with exercise can be easily measured by multiplying the miles by 100. A five mile run = 500 calories. A three mile walk = 300 calories. Using the attributes of the amazing wheel improves efficiency. Cycling is 33 calories per mile. Skating is 50 calories per mile. There are other ways to burn calories too.

As I am lecturing I am frequently asked, "What is the best form of exercise?" Before giving my answer I will solicit responses from the audience which range from swimming, to cross country skiing, from yoga, to weight lifting. I then tell the audience that I think they are doing something wrong. Exercise that is enjoyable is more likely to be repeated. "Can anyone name a more enjoyable form of exercise than sex?"

- Sex if you are single = 144 calories
- Sex if you are married = 112 calories

I thus recommend sex done like you are single but while you are married. It is another example of activity burning calories.

But doctor, you say, "I don't know how much I am moving or how far I am walking. My last doctor said to get 30 minutes of exercise." The government and health agencies will give this same instruction to exercise for an amount of time as well. It is a mostly useless suggestion. I have patients that will travel only ½ mile (50 calories) in thirty minutes. I have other patients that will travel over 6 miles in that same time (600 calories). Measure your exercise in terms of calories burned and the data will become useful.

Now, back to Lawrence's watch. It is possible to burn 2000 calories playing basketball. As this activity is done on foot it would require the same amount of work as running twenty miles (2000 calories/100 calories per mile =20 miles). Running twenty miles is significantly more work than playing basketball for 2 hours like we are playing basketball. Our work rate on the court is similar to a run at a pace of ten minute miles. That would put the calorie burn at 1200 calories (120 minutes/1 mile per ten minutes = 12 miles; 12 miles = 1200 calories). This is a big difference from what the watch reports. *Caveat emptor* (buyer beware).

The errant data from exercise equipment can make it much more challenging to navigate weight management. There are 3600 calories in a pound of fat. This is not just my fat and your fat, which is to say, human fat. The pint of olive oil beside my stove has 3600 calories in the bottle. The pint of coconut oil has 3600 calories as well. A pound of the truffle oil that I love has 3600 calories as well. A pound of lard (pig fat) is the same too.

I find the 3600 calories depressing and amazing. Amazing because we can store the ability to walk 36 miles in one pound of flesh (3600/100 calories per mile=36 miles). Depressing because we have to walk 36 miles to burn one pound of fat. Amazing because we can ride a bicycle over 100 miles (3600/33 calories per mile=109 miles) on a pound of fat. Depressing because we can ride a bicycle 100 miles and still not have burned a full pound of fat.

These amazing, depressing 3600 calories help to explain some things. "Doctor, I have worked out every day for 30 minutes for two weeks and I still have not lost any weight!" Well, the 200 calories you have burned each day during your workout would burn off a pound a fat in 18 days (3600/200 calories per day = 18 days). I say "would" because it often does not actually happen. And the odds are worse for women (sorry, you just tend to eat more after exercising). And it is very frustrating. It is so frustrating people give up.

Do not give up. Knowing it will take 18 days at your current effort level may be of some help. Also of some help may be the likely fact you are eating more as you exercise more. It does not take much extra food to wipe away all of your hard work. Fourteen corn chips will do it. One pint of soda will do it. And that is the other side of the formula.

Here is the mathematical formula for a stable waist size:

Calories Consumed = Calories Burned

This may seem boring or overwhelming but it is very important for your success. Let's break down each component beginning with the calories consumed side of the equation.

It is useful for purposes of both thought and math to look at calories consumed on a day-by-day basis. Longer periods of time are more telling (say calories consumed over the course of a year compared to the calories burned over the same year) but the math involved in looking at 803,000 calories is beyond our scope. So we will take things one day at a time. One day at a time is not too difficult.

Calories Consumed =
everything you eat + everything you drink

Or

Calories Per Day = Breakfast + Creamer in Your Coffee + Lunch + Afternoon Snack + Dinner

- 2 eggs = 140 calories
- 2 slices toast = 200 calories
- 1 tbsp butter for said toast = 100 calories
- Coffee = 0 calories
- 2 tbsp creamer = 100 calories
- Turkey sandwich = 340 calories
- 1 bag chips = 140 calories
- Granola bar = 100 calories
- Spaghetti = 400 calories
- Salad = 40 calories
- Salad dressing = 140 calories
- Ice cream = 300 calories

Total = 2000 calories

Calories burned = basal metabolic rate + all of your activity (thinking and blinking, walking and talking, chewing and spitting).

- Basal rate = 1200 calories
- 3 mile walk = 300 calories
- Fidgeting with a pen and bouncing your knee while in a meeting = 12 calories
- Taking the stairs = 16 calories
- Taking the elevator = 3 calories
- Changing the channel on the TV in 1970 = 2 calories
- Changing the channel with your remote = 0.1 calories

- Shivering at the bus stop for 10 minutes after you forgot your jacket = 300 calories
- Brushing your teeth = 3 calories
- Chewing your daily bread = 30 calories
- Vigorous married person sex = 140 calories

Total = 2000 calories

Most people understand the idea of this in general terms but there are commonly misplaced ideas.

1) People underestimate how many calories they are eating.
2) People overestimate how many calories they burn with exercise.
3) People don't grasp that the major determinant of calorie burn is by basal metabolic rate.
4) People take days off or think they deserve a "treat" or "reward." The fact that it is your birthday or anniversary does not change the calorie content in a piece of pie. One extra food reward on six special days a year will lead to one pound of weight gain in a year. If your celebrations include a special drink and a special desert then you are probably looking at two pounds a year. Twenty pounds in a decade.

Any of the mistakes above can lead to failure. Making myriad of the above mistakes, which is common, makes it very difficult to be successful in weight management. The food industry makes it even harder and we will explore that in the next science lesson.

Chapter: 13

A Word from Our Sponsor

"Call to Me, and I will answer you, and show you great and mighty things" Jeremiah 33:3

I love cooking. I like shopping for the food. I like dreaming of combining the items in the pantry and refrigerator into something beautiful. I learned from my grandmother. She never used a recipe so I don't either. This creates some very unique meals. In fact, because I can't make the same thing twice, all of the meals at our house are unique. But, while I love cooking, I don't really like the cleaning part. To minimize any cleaning associated with cooking I use as few pots, pans, and dishes as possible. I was particularly efficient at this prior to getting married. Meat and vegetables onto the grill and then eaten directly off of the grill with a knife and fork. The grill was simply left to be scraped with the next use and the knife and fork were placed in the dishwasher. Cleanup time was less than one minute.

The use of dishes while eating was of more work than importance to me. The 'Man' was not going to bring me down by making me use a plate that I did not want to use just because it was convention. I had the system beaten. And then I got married. Using plates and not eating over the grill or sink was an unanticipated area for compromise in our marriage. I could have seen it coming had I thought about it, but it never crossed my mind. Amy likes to use lots of dishes and actually sit down at a table to eat the food. This means more cleaning. While I don't really like cleaning, I do like a happy wife, so bring on the dish soap.

One evening about five years down the path leading to Jesus, the kids were in bed and Amy was at work. I was doing the dishes. Usually while doing the dishes I listen to very loud rock-n-roll. Not loud enough to make an eardrum bleed, but loud enough to make the house shake. That night, so as not to disturb dreaming dumplings, the music was off. I began to contemplate theology. I had prayed many times to accept Jesus and for the forgiveness of my sins. But, I still had all of these doubts. I still did not believe fully. I wondered how to know if I was reconciled with God. Scrub. Slosh. Squeek. Clink.

I came to the conclusion that I may really only know after death, and as suicide may complicate the reconciliation picture, then the answer may be a few years away. So I prayed. "God, if I were to die right now, would I go to heaven?" Something unique and unforgettable happened. I felt a sense of warmth, comfort, and absolute peace enter me. It was more powerful than love or lust or hate. I was given an answer from God. Absolute peace. Answered prayer.

I had never experienced anything like it. I am not sure how long it lasted as time seemed to stop. It was so powerful that even while it was happening I was wondering what possible combination of neurotransmitters could produce such a severe experience. Maybe a drug overdose and a seizure at the same time? While not as public or as severe as Saul's blindness on the road to Damascus, it was just as meaningful to me.

A few things became evident to my skeptical self as a result of this. First, answered prayer exists, which also implies that God exists and that He cares and is interactive. Second, there was a great sense of peace regarding my reconciliation with God. Third, I was angry that it had taken my entire life to hear from God. The entire long arduous process would have been so much easier if God would have just started speaking to me at the beginning. I mean, what was the point of all of that hard work? Well, a few things come to mind on that count.

I wish I had heard the gospel and simply believed. It would have been much easier and joyous and peaceful. But, then I would not be very useful from an apologetics perspective. I have the ability as a result of my hard work to have discourse on challenging issues surrounding faith. If I had not put that work in myself, then I would not have the same tools or ability to do this.

In addition, it is possible that had my prayer life been stronger that I would have been more attuned to hearing from God much sooner. As exemplified by this book, God has continued to answer prayer since that time in my kitchen. As exemplified by this book, I have not always liked the answer to prayer or the call that God gives. And, as you may have grasped by now, I am stubborn and don't always do things the first time I am told. For God I should. I am forever indebted to God for the completely graceful gift of Jesus. But, I am also human and sinful and that is often modeled as stubbornness. It is not just with God either. Amy will happily agree that I am stubborn in other areas as well. Unfortunately, stubbornness is not the worst of my sins.

Chapter: 14

Science Lesson # 7 – Food Labels and Marketing

"Like a dog that returns to its vomit is a fool that returns to his folly." Proverbs 26:11

One of my favorite marketing slogans came from Jolt Cola: "All of the sugar and twice the caffeine." The company advertised high-sugar high-caffeine soda. If you wanted a jolt to your system, Jolt was there to help you. Unfortunately for Jolt, this marketing strategy proved poor and the company went bankrupt. While I liked the marketing, I never actually bought the drink. After all, it couldn't actually be good for you. And remember, I do not want to get fat.

Hundreds of billions of dollars are spent each year on marketing and marketing research. For instance, car companies know that people will pay a lot more to drive a hybrid car, but only if it says "hybrid" on the car. If that label is removed, or not offered, then the desire to buy the car is removed as well. This is an example of competitive altruism. I wonder, if altruism is competitive, is it really altruistic?

The term "organic" is another one that people are willing to pay a premium for. This is despite the fact that there is no data to prove that eating organic food is actually better for you. There are plenty of good reasons why organic food should be better for us to eat, but studies proving such a benefit do not exist. In fact, a Stanford University meta-analysis on this topic released in the Annals of Internal Medicine in 2012 reviewed every study done on organic food from 1966 to 2011 and found no benefit to organic food. Why then will people pay double or triple for an organic apple? Because they want to. Why do they want to? Because they think it is better for them. Why do they think it is better for them? Because of marketing. Remember, we are willing to pay top dollar for hope.

Now marketing plays a role in almost everything we buy. To think that we are smarter than the marketing machine is naïve. We all have to make choices and while being well-informed helps, there is not a way to escape marketing influence. They even market specifically to people who want to avoid marketing tactics.

Let's review some common marketing practices that food companies use to try to sway you to buy their product. Often they try to trick you into thinking their product is good for you when it is actually harmful. Let's start with the term "sugar free".

Sugar is bad for you right? So sugar free must be good for you right? There are lots of things that are sugar free or "no sugar added." Steak and lobster, popcorn and peanuts, coffee and tea, and chicken and the other white meat are all sugar free. But they are not advertised this way. Advertising them as such would probably make you less likely to buy them. "Sugar free fish only $7.99 a pound" does not sound like fish I would buy.

Foods that will be advertised as sugar free are foods that taste sweet. You would expect them to have sugar in them, and would be very pleased to learn that they did not. Sugar free jelly and sugar free ice cream and sugar free candy and sugar free soda would all be examples where sugar free would sound appealing. This is where you will see the "sugar free" marketing.

These sugar free foods still taste sweet. And they have fewer calories. What is not to like? The answer lies in why they still taste sweet despite having no sugar. All food advertised as sugar free is sweetened with artificial sweetener. If you are still under the impression that artificial sweetener is a good idea, please go back and read chapter two on artificial sweeteners again. While the marketing says "sugar free," what you should read is, "these products will double your risk of diabetes, obesity, high blood pressure, and high cholesterol." If it tastes sweet but does not have an appropriate number of calories, leave it on the shelf.

If sugar is bad for you, then fat must be really bad for you. Therefore "fat free" foods should be a safe choice right? "Fat free" has been around longer than "sugar free" as a marketing slogan. It sure sounds appealing. Free things are good. Fat is bad. "Fat free" must then be very good. While only foods that you would expect to be sweet are advertised as sugar free, any food group may be advertised as "fat free". I have seen fat free bread, licorice, cheese, pasta, milk, coffee cream, candy, and even butter.

But, "fat free" almost always means high carbohydrate. Fat tastes good. A well-marbled fatty steak tastes better than a very lean steak. If the fat is taken out, food does not taste as good. As a palatable alternative, food producers add more carbohydrate to improve the taste.

Let's examine a food label. Note that the label gives information on serving size, calorie content, and three of the four food groups: fat, carbs, and protein.

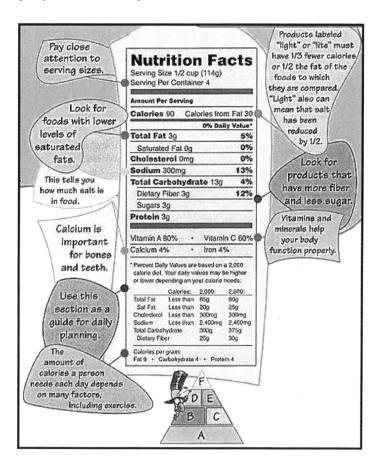

While this is great information, I recommend against eating food that comes with a food label. The food that God made does not have a label on it. I think it is best to eat food that has to be picked or killed. Think of all of the wonderful food available in the Garden of Eden and stick to that. But, if you are going to eat food that has a label, the information provided is helpful.

The first thing to look at is the serving size. This is another place where the marketers will try to trick you. Foods and drinks may be labeled as "100 calories per serving." You would imagine that eating the serving would then be 100 calories. But you would be wrong. What you assume to be a serving may actually be four servings. You must look at the serving size and the number of servings per package.

Perhaps you have had the experience of finding an opened and partially consumed can of soda in the refrigerator. Men do not do this. We know that if you are thirsty enough to open the soda, then you consider it a single serving and you finish the entire can. Most 12 oz. cans are a single serving (there are many exceptions to this with energy drinks, juice, and coffee drinks). When you move up to the 16 oz. or larger size however, typically the food label will determine that there is more than one serving in the bottle. But, it still is packaged like a single serving, just a pleasantly larger single serving. If there are two servings in the package or bottle and you consume the entire thing, you must double all of the other metrics on the label.

Now back to the issue of "fat free." There are two basic tricks that are played in this setting. The first is that the food is not actually fat free, but since the serving size is so small (less than one gram of fat per serving) the FDA does not require reporting it. An example of this is fat free cooking spray.

Nutrition Facts

Serving Size 1/4 sec spray (0.25g)
Servings Per Container About 680

Amount Per Serving

Calories 0   Calories from Fat 0

% Daily Value*

Total Fat 0g	**0%**
Sat Fat 0g	**0%**
Trans Fat 0g	
Polyunsat Fat 0g	
Monounsat Fat 0g	
Cholesterol 0mg	**0%**
Sodium 0mg	**0%**
Total Carb. 0g	**0%**
Protein 0g	**0%**

Not a significant source of dietary fiber, sugars, vitamin A, vitamin C, calcium and iron.

*Percent Daily Values are based on a 2,000 calorie diet

INGREDIENTS: VEGETABLE OIL BLEND* (CANOLA, SOY AND OLIVE OILS), SOY LECITHIN, GRAIN ALCOHOL (PERSERVATIVE), DIMETHYLPOLYSILOXANE AND PROPELLANT.
CONTAINS: SOY
*ADDS A TRIVIAL AMOUNT OF FAT

Owned & Distributed by:
GFA BRANDS, INC.
Paramus, NJ 07652-1432
201-421-3970
Visit: www.smartbalance.com

DIRECTIONS:
SHAKE WELL. Point arrow on button towards red mark on can. Hold can upright 6-12 inches away. Spray onto unheated cook/ bakeware or grill.

©2012
GFA Brands, Inc.
All rights reserved

As you can see, the only ingredient is oil. Oil is fat. Pure fat. A can of six ounce cooking spray contains 170 grams of fat for a total of 1570 calories (170 grams * 9 calories per gram of fat). How can 1570 calories of pure fat be "fat free?" And who gets 680 uses out of a can of cooking spray? Well, the serving size is so small that the FDA will allow the company to falsely market the food as "fat free". The same trick is used with trans-fats. There are many products that contain small amounts of hydrogenated oil. The amount is small enough that they are allowed to call the product "trans-fat free." I am not at all happy about this trickery. If you took just the first drag of cigarette after cigarette, would you be allowed to say that you don't smoke?

The more common trick with "fat free" is that it means high carbohydrate. Take a look at the carbohydrate content on "fat free" foods:

Nutrition Facts	
Serving Size ½ cup (125 g)	
Servings Per Container 3	
Amount Per Serving	
Calories 100	Calories from Fat 10
	% Daily Value*
Total Fat 4g	7%
Saturated Fat 0g	0%
Cholesterol 0mg	0%
Sodium 250mg	10%
Potassium 530mg	15%
Total Carbohydrate 8g	3%
Dietary Fiber 1g	4%
Sugars 7g	
Protein 8g	

Nutrition Facts	
Serving Size ½ cup (125 g)	
Servings Per Container 3	
Amount Per Serving	
Calories 152	Calories from Fat 0
	% Daily Value*
Total Fat 0g	0%
Saturated Fat 0g	0%
Cholesterol 0mg	0%
Sodium 250mg	10%
Potassium 530mg	15%
Total Carbohydrate 30g	10%
Dietary Fiber 1g	4%
Sugars 29g	
Protein 8g	

As you can see, foods that are marketed to you as being good for you because they are fat free are often otherwise not good for you because they are high carb. It is fine if you want to eat candy or pretzels or other high carbohydrate foods. Just don't deluded yourself into thinking they are good for you in any way because they are "fat free." As with "sugar free," foods labeled "fat free" are probably not a good idea.

The Atkin's Diet has been one of the most popular diets in my lifetime. The general idea is to remove all carbohydrate from the diet initially, and then re-introduce some to maintain weight when a goal weight is reached. The diet works well for weight loss. That probably is why it has been popular. Interestingly, every study that has been done on the Atkin's Diet shows that people's cholesterol actually improves despite eating gobs of bacon and cheese. It seems that *being* fat is harder on the cholesterol level than *eating* fat. We'll look more at the Atkin's Diet and the effect of carbohydrates on hunger and metabolism in the chapter 16.

Given the popularity of this diet, the marketing geniuses began to market foods as "low carb." The idea here is that if eating low carb leads to weight loss, then "low carb" will attract buyers willing to pay a premium. Regular beef jerky costs 99 cents. Low carb beef jerky costs $1.29. It is the same food, just different marketing. All beef jerky is low carb because all meat is low carb.

I would like to mention here that there are only four sources of calories. I think of these sources as my four food groups: Carbohydrate (carbs), protein, fat, and alcohol. Most of the foods eaten by humans are mostly carbohydrate. If you pick it, it is most likely a carbohydrate. Fruits and vegetables are almost pure carbohydrate. If you can kill it, then it is mostly protein. Fats come from seeds, nuts, animals, and some vegetables. Alcohol is the excrement of yeast that has been chewing on carbohydrate. Thank you, yeast.

This notion of food composition is helpful in wisely discerning the low carb marketing. If it is killed it is already low carb so that is just telling you what you should already know. The "low carb" marketing should perk your interest however when it pertains to a food that should be carbohydrate rich. Any food that is sweet should be carbohydrate rich as it is carb, and carb alone, that creates a sweet taste naturally. Additionally, any food that is starchy should be carbohydrate rich as carb is the only source of starch. Therefore, if you see a sweet or starchy food that is labeled "low carb" then you should check the label for artificial sweeteners. That is the only way to make a sweet food "low carb." Again, refer back to chapter two if you need a refresher on artificial sweeteners.

Next let's discuss the "25% less" marketing. This marketing is clearly directed at people trying to make wise choices when purchasing food. Twenty-five precent fewer calories and 25% less sugar claims are easy to find at the store. The thinking is along the lines of sugar is bad, so 25% less sugar is good. I will make this one easy for you. If it claims to have 25% less, it is bad for you. Always.

If you want "25% less", then just buy or eat 25% less. Please do not be tricked into buying chocopuffies just because they have 25% less sugar. Please do not be tricked into buying double stuffed double chunk cookies that have 25% fewer calories. An advertising slogan of "pay for the whole bag of apples, but we will only give you 75%" would not sell many apples. The "25% less" advertising is the same thing. If you are going to eat fudge, eat the real stuff, enjoy it, and get your money's worth. Then work those calories off.

Another common marketing slogan is "whole grain." Whole grains are good for you (unless you are type 2 diabetic). As whole grains are good for you, then foods labeled as "whole grain" should be good for you right? The answer unfortunately is that it depends. It depends on if the food is actually whole grain. Most of the foods labeled a "whole grain" have whole grain in them. If they did not then it would be another example of lying, as was discussed when foods labeled "fat free or trans-fat free." In this setting the labeling is only misleading.

All foods labeled "whole grain" do in fact contain some whole grain. The problem is that most of the foods labeled in this fashion contain mostly refined and processed grains with an added pinch of whole grain. It is brilliant marketing. It allows the food manufacturers to make foods that are as pleasing to the palate as processed grain foods while tricking you into buying them, often at a higher price, because you think they are better for you.

I enjoy being tricked in the surprise party or magician sort of way. I don't like being tricked when it means that I am getting ripped-off. I place this "whole grain" trick in the rip-off category. You can only determine if the marketing is real or a rip-off by looking at the ingredients. Here are three examples of breads that were each labeled as "whole grain":

Healthy Life Original 100% Whole Wheat Whole Grain Bread

Nutrition Facts

Serving Size 2 Slices (41g)
Servings Per Container 11

Amount Per Serving	%DV	2 Slice	1 Slice
Calories 70		Calories from Fat 5	
Calories 35		Calories from Fat 0	

	% Daily Value*	2 Slice	1 Slice
Total Fat 0g,0g		0%	0%
Saturated Fat 0g,0g		0%	0%
Trans Fat 0g,0g			
Polyunsaturated Fat 0g,0g			
Monounsaturated Fat 0g,0g			
Cholesterol 0mg,0mg		0%	0%
Sodium 150mg,80mg		6%	3%
Total Carbohydrate 16g,8g		5%	3%
Dietary Fiber 5g,3g		20%	12%
Sugars 2g,1g			
Protein 5g,2g			

Vitamin A 0% 0%		Vitamin C 0% 0%	
Calcium 10% 4%		Iron 4% 2%	
Thiamin 6% 4%		Riboflavin 2% 2%	
Niacin 6% 2%		Folic Acid 2% 0%	

* Percent Daily Values (DV) are based on a 2,000 calorie diet. Your daily values may be higher or lower depending on your calorie needs:

	Calories:	2,000	2,500
Total Fat	Less than	65g	80g
Sat Fat	Less than	20g	25g
Cholesterol	Less than	300mg	300mg
Sodium	Less than	2,400mg	2,400mg
Total Carbohydrate		300g	375g
Dietary Fiber		25g	30g

NO Bromate
NO Hydrogenated Oil
0 Grams *Trans* Fats
NO Saturated Fats
NO Cholesterol

INGREDIENTS: WATER, 100% WHOLE GRAIN WHOLE WHEAT FLOUR, SOY FIBER AND/OR WHEAT FIBER AND/OR SUGAR CANE FIBER, WHEAT GLUTEN, YEAST, BROWN SUGAR, CONTAINS 2% OR LESS OF THE FOLLOWING: MOLASSES, SALT, DOUGH CONDITIONERS (MONO & DIGLYCERIDES, SODIUM STEAROYL LACTYLATE, ETHOXYLATED MONO- DIGLYCERIDES, ASCORBIC ACID, CALCIUM PEROXIDE, AZODICARBONAMIDE), CALCIUM PROPIONATE (TO PREVENT SPOILAGE), GUAR GUM, YEAST NUTRIENTS (CALCIUM SULFATE, CALCIUM CARBONATE, AMMONIUM SULFATE), FUMARIC ACID, WHEAT STARCH, PALM OIL, SOY LECITHIN.
CONTAINS: WHEAT, SOY.

LEWIS BAKERIES, INC.
GENERAL OFFICES: EVANSVILLE, IN 47710

Allergy Advisory: Produced on the same bakery equipment as baked goods containing milk, eggs, or nuts. Therefore, this product may inadvertently contain milk, eggs, or nuts to which some people may be allergic.

While we make every effort to post the most current product nutrition facts and ingredients on this web site, your best source of product information is what is printed on the package you purchase.

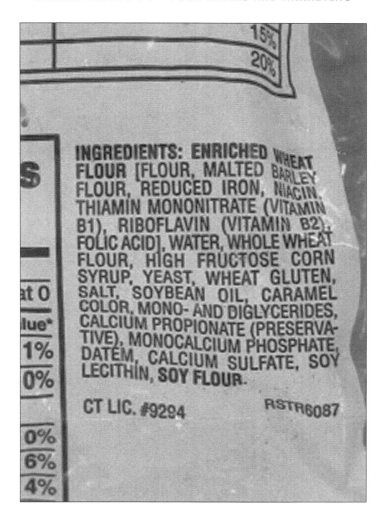

INGREDIENTS: ENRICHED WHEAT FLOUR [FLOUR, MALTED BARLEY FLOUR, REDUCED IRON, NIACIN, THIAMIN MONONITRATE (VITAMIN B1), RIBOFLAVIN (VITAMIN B2), FOLIC ACID], WATER, WHOLE WHEAT FLOUR, HIGH FRUCTOSE CORN SYRUP, YEAST, WHEAT GLUTEN, SALT, SOYBEAN OIL, CARAMEL COLOR, MONO- AND DIGLYCERIDES, CALCIUM PROPIONATE (PRESERVATIVE), MONOCALCIUM PHOSPHATE, DATEM, CALCIUM SULFATE, SOY LECITHIN, **SOY FLOUR.**

CT LIC. #9294   RSTR6087

Nutrition Facts
Serving Size 1 Slice (54g)
Servings Per Container Approx. 13

Amount Per Serving

Calories 130 — Calories from Fat 15

	%Daily Value*
Total Fat 1.5g	2%
Saturated Fat 0g	0%
Trans Fat 0g	
Cholesterol 0mg	0%
Sodium 250mg	10%
Total Carbohydrate 24g	8%
Dietary Fiber 2g	7%
Sugars 1g	
Protein 6g	

Vitamin A 0%	•	Vitamin C	0%
Calcium 2%	•	Iron	10%

* Percent Daily Values are based on a 2,000 calorie diet. Your daily values may be higher or lower depending on your calorie needs:

		Calories:	2,000	2,500
Total Fat	Less than		65g	80g
Saturated Fat	Less than		20g	25g
Cholesterol	Less than		300mg	300mg
Sodium	Less than		2,400mg	2,400mg
Total Carbohydrate			300g	375g
Dietary Fiber			25g	30g

Calories per gram:
Fat 9 • Carbohydrate 4 • Protein 4

INGREDIENTS: ENRICHED BLEACHED FLOUR (WHEAT FLOUR, MALTED BARLEY FLOUR, ASCORBIC ACID, NIACIN, IRON, THIAMINE, RIBOFLAVIN, FOLIC ACID), WATER, SOURDOUGH STARTER, MULTIGRAIN MIX (SUNFLOWER SEEDS, SESAME SEEDS, CRACKED WHEAT, BARLEY, RYE, TRITICALE, MILLET, OATS, CORN, BROWN RICE, FLAX SEEDS), BUCKWHEAT FLOUR, SALT, SOY LECITHIN, SOY FLOUR. NO PRESERVATIVES ADDED.

As you can see the ingredient list is similar. You can also see that each bread contains whole grain. In example A the first ingredient is 100% whole wheat. In examples B and C, however, the first ingredient is wheat flour (that means refined/processed) and the whole grain does not show up until the third or fourth ingredient. As food ingredients are listed in order of decreasing content we can know there is more whole wheat than salt, but not likely much more. Bread B adds caramel coloring to make the bread look more "whole grain". Bread A is honest bread. I would buy bread A. Bread B and C are rip-off bread and I boycott all rip-off foods.

Seeing "whole grain" on the front of a label should serve as a cue to look at the ingredient list. If the first ingredient is not 100% whole such-and-such (wheat, oats, rye, barley, amaranth, millet, buckwheat, spelt, corn, brown rice, or triticale) then it is not actually whole grain food.

Advertisers and marketers are geniuses. They are smarter than me and they are smarter than you. My hope is that by enlightening you to some of the common marketing tricks you will be harder prey to catch. I thought about including information of "gluten free" and "organic" in this section as well, but I want to avoid hate mail. People love their gluten free cinnamon rolls and their organic frosted toasties cereal. I will have to save those for a book written under a pseudonym.

Chapter: 15

And Then I Learned I Am a Sinner

"You shall have no other gods before me."
"You shall not make for yourself a carved image,
or any likeness of anything that is in heaven
above, or that is in the earth beneath, or that is
in the water under the earth. You shall not bow
down to them or serve them...." Exodus 20:3-5

When Amy and I were pregnant with our first child, we (like all expectant parents) began to contemplate names. I liked Stanley. My friend Dan's dad was named Stanley and he was an admirable combination of being a man's man and a kind person at the same time. You were pretty sure he had killed people, but if you needed help, he would drop everything to give it to you. Amy thought Stanley was too "old" sounding. Amy liked Quinton. I pointed out that as this means fifth child it was not really appropriate for our first child. We moved from the 1001 baby names book to the much larger 10,001 baby names book. Amy read it cover to cover. We also looked through scripture to see if a name would jump out at us. Adam felt too generic. Gomer and Kenaniah were too defining. Amy said, "What about Jonah?"

I like the name Jonah just fine. But, I am not too fond of Jonah the prophet. Made of just four chapters and comprising two pages of my Bible, Jonah is a short book. Most people, including children, are familiar with the story. A prophet of God is swallowed by a great fish. But that is not the heart of the story.

Jonah is really about revealing human nature. My nature. Your nature. It is also about revealing God's nature. Jonah was called by God to go to the wicked city of Nineveh. He did not go. He ran the other direction. This is one of the reasons I am not fond of Jonah. I think that if God tells you to do something you should just do it. God clearly wants Jonah to do this work so he creates a storm and lets Jonah sit in the stinking stomach of a giant fish for three days to contemplate things. After the ride in the fish, Jonah goes to Nineveh. He prophesies there and the people repent and are saved.

Jonah becomes more unlikable here as he is exceedingly displeased at God's choice to show love and mercy to the wicked Assyrians. Jonah does not like God's nature. Jonah is so angry that he wishes for God to take his life.

At this point God tries to teach Jonah a lesson by having a kikayon plant, which Jonah did not plant or create, grow out of the ground and give Jonah some shade. Jonah likes the plant but then God sends a worm to kill it, and it withers. Jonah is hot from the sun and so angry about the plant that he again asks to die. God confronts him on this by asking Jonah if his pity over the plant, which he did not labor over, which came into being in a night and perished in a night, was justified. For if Jonah could care that much for a plant, should God not care for the 120,000 citizens of Nineveh?

No, Jonah is not likable in this story. And we never learn if God's message to Jonah sinks in as the story ends abruptly at that point. What would cause Jonah to act this way? What would cause him to fail to follow God's will, and then to be so angry about God showing mercy that he would wish to die over it? I have a good idea, because it turns out that I am like Jonah.

After my divine interaction experience while doing the dishes things hummed along nicely. I had a wife that I love and kids that were easier to love as each month passed (I was not too fond of the baby stage, I prefer playing to ogling). I had a job that I loved, and was attending a church that I loved. All the while I was being loved by my wife, my kids, my parents (who live a few miles away), my in-laws (who live even closer), and my patients. I had it great. Unfortunately, I also had an under-appreciation for the gospel.

The reason for this under-appreciation was that I really did not feel very sinful. I treated everyone well. I did not have any vices except exercise. I was doing churchly things like service team, Bible study, growth group, getting food to the poor, etc. I was doing God's work at my work, praying with patients, praying with staff, and seeking His will constantly (unless I was too busy which was often).

It was not as though I thought I was sinless. I had impure thoughts. I did not cherish my wife as consistently as I would like. I was often angry. My children still make me angry frequently. And it is the self-interested type, not the righteous type of anger. Also, there were opportunities for service or reaching out to someone and I let them pass for no other reason than I did not really feel like it at the time. No, I did not feel sinless, just much less sinful than average. Perhaps you behave well and feel this way too. It may well be easier for the murderer to see the depth of the gospel than it was for me. And then I learned what a rotten sinner I really am. I will say it had been hidden in plain sight, and I was just blind to it.

I did not understand idolatry. I had the idea that idolatry meant worshiping a carved image, a golden calf, a false god. Idolatry is that, but not just. Idolatry is elevating anything above God or His will. It is excessive worship of something that is not God. Although God took care to warn us twice, with the first two of the Ten Commandments, I still missed it. Idolatry is what led to the first sin. Adam and Eve ate of the fruit because they were elevating their will above the will of God. Every sin since that original one has happened for the same reason. Jonah's original lack of obedience, and then petulance after God was merciful, were likewise elevations of his will above God's will. At the heart of it, Jonah believed that his own sense of justice was better than God's. It was idolatry that made Jonah flee to Tarshish and it was idolatry that had him so angry when God was merciful and saved the sinners in Nineveh. Imagine Jonah's response to Jesus, who likewise spent three days in the belly of hell, and came to save those who did not deserve it.

I don't think you will find it any stretch of the imagination to see that adultery, murder, thievery, lying, covetousness, blasphemy, and failing to honor one's parents are all examples of things that occur as a result of elevating something above the will of God. God teaches not to steal, but you want the thing more than you want to follow the will of God, so you steal. God teaches forgiveness but you are so offended that you elevate your own justice above His will and you hold a grudge (or murder). God teaches faithfulness in a marriage, but you want the taste of someone other than your spouse so you elevate your own will and fornicate. Paul defines covetousness as idolatry in Colossians 3:5. In fact, all of the overt sins of the Ten Commandments are failures of the first two. The problem is, idolatry goes even deeper.

Although I can keep myself from stealing and murdering and fornicating (at least overtly, the Sermon on the Mount brings a deeper level of complexity and conviction here where I am guilty of all ten of the Ten Commandments in a given day), it is harder to keep myself from inappropriately elevating the things I love. I love my wife, my children, exercise, vitality, my job, my financial security, and myself. I habitually elevate the interest of these things above the will of God. And that is idolatry, and it is sinful.

The idols in your life may not be that hard to identify. Make a list of the things, people, ideas, and behaviors that you prioritize over God. I already gave you my list. It is the things I love. I love my wife, my children, exercise, vitality, my job, my financial security, and myself. And I know that I consistently put the interests of these beloved things above the will of God.

The idea that you can love your spouse or kids in an idolatrous (ie sinful) manner may be a stretch for you. Allow me to elaborate. Let us return to the example of a prideful Karl doing his very best to be a good husband. Now, does God like husbands to be good? Yes. But, there is a bit more to it that just that. The how of it is very important. If Karl strives for good husbandry out of his own will (self interest) he may very well be successful. This success leads to pride. If Karl is not successful out of his own will then this produces anxiety or anguish.

Now pretend that instead of trying to be a good husband for himself, Karl strives to be a good husband in order to serve God. Karl is now on assignment and serving God's will. It may not look different to an observer. But it clearly looks different to God. It is also a different experience for Karl. God is involved. There is divine relationship. Karl can pray and ask for help. God sends a helper in the form of his Holy Spirit. Now Karl is serving God with God's help. This is good news. God does not get tired. God does not grow impatient. God does not have desires of the flesh than can damage a marriage. Karl will be a better imperfect husband by serving God than he was by serving his own will.

In addition, the object of this service, in this case Amy, can behave in ways that make Karl less interested in being a good husband. If Amy were to drain the bank account, nag, become addicted to drugs, or have an affair, she would be harder for Karl to want to serve as her husband. Amy behaves poorly so Karl puts forth less effort at husbanding, and now we are on a path to marital strife and eventually divorce. With Karl serving God's will in the marriage instead of his own will the outcome may be very different. Regardless of Amy's behaviors, Karl is called to patience, kindness, slowness to anger, and forgiveness.

In serving the will of Karl the outcomes were pride or anxiety. When Karl instead serves the will of God, things will look different. If his marriage flourishes, Karl will feel joy and give thanks to God. It will be seen as a glorification of God's Kingdom. Because Karl was not working for himself, and also because he was not working alone (because the Holy Spirit is now helping), the pride and self-righteousness do not appear. Now, if we assume that the marriage does not do well, what happens then? Assuming that Karl has been serving the will of God, this implies that a struggling marriage is not Karl's fault. The anguish and anxiety may be absent completely or at least diminished. Circumstances can now be viewed as God's will, which is often beyond human understanding. Or, perhaps suffering, which is clearly an expected part of life in Christ. Recall Romans chapter five:

> *[1] Therefore, since we have been justified through faith, we have peace with God through our Lord Jesus Christ, [2] through whom we have gained access by faith into this grace in which we now stand. And we boast in the hope of the glory of God. [3] Not only so, but we also glory in our sufferings, because we know that suffering produces perseverance; [4] perseverance, character; and character, hope. [5] And hope does not put us to shame, because God's love has been poured out into our hearts through the Holy Spirit, who has been given to us.*

Suffering in God's will is productive. Character and hope are produced in us. Even more important than hope, however, is that we are brought into greater relationship with God as we trust in His will. Seeing your marriage as an assignment from God thus leads to joy, thanksgiving, glorification of God's kingdom, character, hope, and divine relationship. This is clearly a greater outcome than the pride produced by serving one's own will.

A specific example of idolatry in my life looks very similar to Jonah. I prayed for God to show me the work of my hands. God put it upon my heart to write this book in 2008 (Karl, go to Nineveh). I came up with a bunch of really good reasons why that was a bad idea (my will) and tried to stay in Tarshish. As no great fish came to swallow me up, I simply remained in my idolatry for years with God's will on my heart, and me resisting it.

Pastor Charles finally convicted me of my error. He is from Rwanda. After the genocide he was looking at a group of children and babies that had been orphaned by the genocide and felt God was calling him to serve those kids. There were rotting bodies everywhere. He had no way to feed or care for the kids. He had other plans. He wanted to run away to Tarshish. He did not feel adequate for the job God was calling him to, nor did he want to do it. But Pastor Charles did not run. He stayed and saved those kids. And as I listened to Pastor Charles in church in 2011, I was cut to the heart at how I had failed God's command. I began to write that very day.

It was when I realized what a habitual idolizer I am that I began to better appreciate the depth of the gospel. I remain both sinful and convicted in my idolatry. I also remain repentant. I also know that I am completely forgiven and washed clean of all of my sin by God's grace. Thanks be to God.

Chapter: 16

Science Lesson #8 –
The Glycemic Index

"How sweet are your words to my taste, sweeter than honey to my mouth." Psalm 119:103

As a boy raised by Midwestern parents, I did not eat much rice growing up. We would eat Chinese food only occasionally at home. In such cases we would have white rice as part of the meal. My mom liked to make a special dessert after dinner by heavily dusting the rice with sugar and cinnamon. The family assumed this cinnamon-sweet dessert rice to be less good for you given its sugar-coating.

I followed this common knowledge that sugar and fat were probably bad for you in my dietary choices into adulthood. I was working hard at not getting fat, and I was willing to give up sugar and ice cream and butter to make that happen. I will admit that this approach did not always leave me feeling well. If I ate pancakes for breakfast, I would turn quite grouchy by midmorning and I would occasionally feel so woozy that I would pass out while playing sports. I would literally run out of fuel on the field or on the court. Most people would probably ask for a substitute when they started to feel dizzy, weak, and lightheaded. I am too stubborn for that. I would keep running until the lights literally went out. This did not occur after eating an omelet for breakfast. It also kept the wooziness at bay if I ate prior to the game and then again at half-time. But why?

I did not get my answer in medical school. Medical school nutrition covered the Krebs cycle and the number of calories per gram of fat, carb, and protein. Medical school nutrition covered what a cardiac diet or a diabetic diet would look like in the hospital. But it was mostly basic nutrition science. Most of the applied nutrition science I learned on my own by reading nutrition articles and journals. My most despised food group, the artificial sweeteners, achieved that acclaim through reading of such research articles. My favorite food principle also came of this research: the glycemic index.

The glycemic index is a measure of how fast a food turns into glucose in the blood after it is eaten. It is a measure of digestive speed. Now the digestive process is quite complicated, but an understanding of the basics will be helpful.

The first part of the digestive process occurs before the food gets to the mouth. Cleaning and cutting and cooking food is a manner of aiding digestion. Oats that are chewed off of the stalk are much slower to digest than oats that are picked, rolled very flat, pre-cooked, and then dried out and placed in a small brown paper package for you to add water and stir and enjoy. The more processing and cutting and cooking that food has gone through prior to your eating of it, the less work your body has to do to digest the remainder of it.

The next part of the digestive process occurs in the mouth. Food is chewed. This increases the surface area of it to allow for easier absorption. Chewing turns the food on your plate into baby food for your stomach. At the same time an enzyme in spit called amylase begins to rapidly break down starch into glucose. This baby food and glucose mix next hits the stomach where acid breaks down the food into even smaller particles.

These smaller particles then mix with the digestive juices of the liver, gall bladder, and pancreas in the small intestine and are absorbed into the bloodstream. These absorbed nutrients then are transported to the liver for cleaning prior to being sent via the bloodstream to the rest of the body to be used as fuel for our body parts.

The non-digested portions are then moved to the large bowel where water is sucked out. The large bowel then drops this waste product into the porcelain, hopefully without a splash. And the process is finished.

The digestive process for carbohydrates is especially fast. Energy put into the mouth can be available for use in the blood in just a couple of minutes. The measure of just how fast the carbs turn into digested energy is called the glycemic index. This index is a percentage of how fast the food turns into glucose in the blood compared to eating pure glucose (the most easily digested and pure form of sugar).

For example, the glycemic index of white rice is 90. This means that white rice turns into glucose by the digestive process and is available for use 90% as fast as pure glucose is. Rice does not taste sweet. The ability of the body to convert something not sweet into something that is pure sugar energy is astounding. A couple of other glycemic index examples are French baguette = 97, pancakes = 99, baked potato = 100. For these foods you may as well be eating pure glucose as that is what you are dumping into the system. Note that I did not say "may as well be eating sugar." Table sugar is sucrose. Sucrose has a glycemic index of 65.

Well, how can it be that sugar is digested into glucose slower than a potato? It has to do with the bonds that hold the carbohydrate together. Starches like bread, rice, potato, carrots, and grains are formed of row after row of glucose molecules. This starch bond is very easily broken apart by the enzyme in spit called amylase. By the time the starch hits the stomach much of it is already broken down into glucose.

Sucrose by comparison tastes sweet. Sucrose is made of a glucose molecule bonded to a fructose molecule. This bond cannot be broken by spit. It can be broken by acid however. The acid in the stomach does the job. Once the glucose and fructose are cleaved apart by the stomach acid the glucose is rapidly absorbed but the fructose has to be converted in the liver two times before it can be used for energy. These conversions slow the digestive process significantly. So much so that fructose has a glycemic index of 19 which is the lowest of all of the sugars. In summary, table sugar is digested much slower than starchy foods.

The sugar that my mom used to add to the white rice was actually slowing down how fast the rice would be metabolized. The same is true of the syrup on pancakes. Pancakes have a glycemic index of 99. Maple syrup is 56 and Mrs. Butterworths and other syrup brands that are made from high fructose corn syrup have a glycemic index of 64. It would be common to think or hear, "Oh dear, don't add too much syrup to your waffle." But instead, you would be better off skipping the pancake and just drinking the syrup.

Pure starches have no redemptive nutritional value. The label on the white rice at my house has 0% of vitamins, calcium, or iron. There is no fat and no cholesterol. Just 40 grams of pure starch per ¼ cup. While I would market this product as being "fat free, cholesterol free, sugar free, and no high-fructose corn syrup" (all true), the lack of any other stuff in starchy foods combined with their high glycemic index of digestion explains the effect that they have on the body.

Chinese food has a reputation of leaving one hungry again two hours after it is eaten. Pancakes are the same. The glycemic index explains this. For a cell in the body to have energy it has to get glucose out of the bloodstream. The body releases insulin as a hormone that informs the cells of the body to take glucose out of the blood. If no insulin is around the glucose level rises in the blood while the cells starve. This is what happens in juvenile diabetes. Assuming you are not juvenile diabetic, eating a carbohydrate (or an artificial sweetener perhaps) causes insulin release. The insulin made by the human body lasts for about 4 hours in the blood after it is released from the pancreas. If the carbohydrates are digested very quickly then the insulin can last longer than the carbohydrate. This will be the case with all high glycemic index foods. This effect is demonstrated in the following chart:

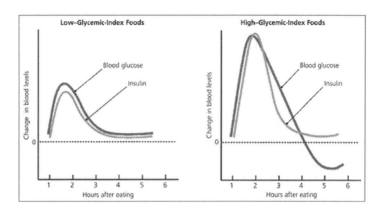

As can be seen, a low glycemic index food will cause a rise in blood sugar and a commensurate rise in insulin. Because the low glycemic index carb is digested slowly, there is a small rise in blood sugar and then a slow return to baseline. In the high glycemic index digestion there is a much higher spike in blood sugar. This leads to a higher spike in insulin. The higher insulin level is bad, in and of itself, as insulin is a growth hormone and makes you fat. The greater problem however is that the insulin lasts longer than the fuel does. This leads to a drop in blood sugar. A low blood sugar produces feelings of anxiety, cold sweat, nausea, irritability, hunger, and eventually collapse. This is exactly what I felt like when dropping to the playing surface after eating pancakes for breakfast. It is also why it is possible to feel hungry so quickly after eating white rice.

This glycemic index knowledge is real power. Sometimes glucose is needed for fuel very quickly in the blood stream. Diabetic can develop low blood sugar from taking too much insulin. A high glycemic index food will kick in very fast to keep them from going into a coma. If an athlete is running out of gas and there is 20 minutes left in the competition, fuel is needed immediately for muscle use. Eating high glycemic index foods in this settings is perfect.

The glycemic index knowledge is also very helpful for the diabetic. In diabetes the sugar (glucose) rises in blood, but the cells are starving because of a signaling problem in getting the glucose into the cell. Patients will often try to avoid sugar as a means to keeping their blood sugar from rising. That approach is not wrong, it is just too narrowly focused. All carbohydrate turns into glucose in the blood. As can be seen with the glycemic index, starches are the most potent at raising blood sugar. Adult diabetes is a carbohydrate metabolism problem, not a sugar problem. The adult diabetic should be limiting carbohydrate intake, especially starches, not just sugar intake.

Most of the time eating food that is digested slowly is preferable. A 2012 article in the *Journal of the American Medical Association* can be added to a compelling list of studies showing that eating a low glycemic index diet is helpful for weight loss and maintenance of weight loss. This article on the effects of calorie composition on energy expenditure suggested that not only does eating fewer rapidly digested carbs help with weight loss, it actually has the metabolism running higher and helps with maintaining weight loss. The higher metabolic rate was equivalent to one hour of moderate intensity exercise per day. This is not surprising to me. As stated previously, insulin makes one fat. Reducing carb intake will reduce insulin levels, and less insulin will make one less fat. This same 2012 *JAMA* article contained an Atkin's Diet arm, and severe carb reduction was even more effective on weight loss than just a low glycemic index diet.

I think that this helps to explain the staying power of popular diets like Atkins (no carb), South Beach (low glycemic index), and medifast (low glycemic index and low carb). (WARNING: The original Atkins and South Beach diets contained no artificial sweeteners. That is no longer the case as both, along with Medifast, are using artificial sweeteners in their proprietary foods, bars, and drinks. Please read chapter two again if you still think that is a good idea.) There is emerging evidence that a calorie is more than just a calorie. Based upon the science, as well as personal experience, as well as the experience of my patients, I recommend a low glycemic index food intake. It takes practice and investigation to learn the glycemic index of foods. The power of that knowledge lasts a lifetime.

Chapter: 17

Idolatry of Food and the Destruction of the Temple

"Therefore God gave them over to the lusts of their hearts, to the dishonoring of their bodies among themselves, because they exchanged the truth about God for a lie and worshiped and served the created rather than the Creator. Who is blessed forever! Amen." Romans 1:24-25

I have a 19-year-old patient named Jeff. Jeff's mom is very concerned about the amount of marijuana that he is smoking. She should be concerned. Jeff smokes weed every day...many times per day if he can afford it. While he feels a little bit guilty about his behavior, he clearly does not feel guilty enough to change. His mom feels defeated and out of options. She has sent him to re-hab, counseling, church, and to a camp for troubled teens. She has loved, punished, pleaded, and prayed. None of this has changed

Jeff's behavior. While Jeff's vice here is pot, the characters and the substance could be changed and the story would still be the same.

I particularly enjoy Thomas Chalmers explanation for behavior that is hard to explain. In his treatise *The Expulsive Power of a New Affection* (readily available online and highly recommended), Chalmers demonstrates that the human heart is always filled with desire, with longing, and with love. If the object of a desire of the heart is removed it will cause pain and will not remove the desire itself. For example, if the desire is work success and the job is removed then retirement will not go well until it either comes to an end (death or a new job), or the affection itself is expulsed from the heart. The only way to expulse a desire is to replace it. Simply trying to remove it does not work. Chalmers states that a void in the heart cannot exist. It must always be full. The question is with what should one fill it?

Jeff has chosen to fill a void in his heart with a drug. He has thus become a slave to his heart's desire. His mom wants him to stop smoking pot, but as Chalmers has stated, that just won't work until Jeff is able to replace the desire for weed with something his heart desires more. This leads to two questions: 1) What caused the void in Jeff's heart that he filled with a drug in the first place? The answer to that may help to give guidance to the answer of the second question. 2) What can expulse his desire for the drug?

The answer to question one, what causes voids in the human heart, can be answered both specifically and generally. In this case Jeff was not helpful in answering. He mostly gazed off into the distance with sleepy eyes. Jeff's mom however had insight instantly. Jeff's dad left them shortly before he started smoking so much weed. Being abandoned by a father would clearly leave a hole in the heart.

John Calvin states the more general sense well when he wrote, "The human heart is a factory of idols...Everyone of us is, from his mother's womb, expert in inventing idols." We are created with a vast capacity to love. Unfortunately we choose to love the things of creation instead of the Creator. Again, think of what occupies your heart. It may be a sports team, the internet, children, romance, the environment, the republic, your job, or any other part of creation. If that is elevated above the will of God, then it is an idol. And you are free to worship it because of free will.

The idols that will be the hardest to remove are those that give sense of purpose and meaning in life. In general, drugs and alcohol and violence do not do this. Those are only superficial symptoms of a deeper problem. It is the places where we get our self-worth in creation that will have the biggest and deepest hooks in our heart. I get a sense of self-worth from being good at my job, from being fit, and from being a good father and husband. It is easy to imagine how people sin when they are sinned against. Provocation leads to retaliation. Hurt feelings lead to withholding love, withholding kindness, and withholding sexual affection. You hurt me so I will hurt you back. Unfortunately, not only do we sin after we have been sinned against, we also sin in response to blessings.

The things that give me value, my blessings, cause me to sin as well. I become judgmental of people who struggle with their weight. I become prideful and full of myself that I am good at my job. It makes me judgmental of parents who don't try as hard or have less gifted children. I may judge those who don't have my same keen level of political insight or value of the environment. Valuing the blessing instead of the Blesser is just another way we commit idolatry. This leads to strange behavior as well. It will lead us to think more highly of people because of their beauty, their intelligence, their sports prowess, their height, or their full set of their own teeth at age 85. This is idolatry at a societal level. While beauty and smarts and speed and teeth are all good blessings, they are gifts from God, not the yardstick God uses to measure us. We should be grateful for these blessings instead of being judgmental of those who were not similarly gifted.

The Olympics comes every four years and every gold medal winner attributes their success to hard work. Yes, hard work plays a large role. But, where did you get the body that is strong and fast? Where did you get your work ethic? Where did you get the intelligence to outmaneuver your opponent? It is the same place everyone else did, you just happened to be more gifted. Thanks should be not to "my hard work" but to "my wonderful creator."

This idea of our success being rooted in our hard work is pervasive in culture. When a rare counter-example like Tim Tebow comes along it makes international news. This is because we are accustomed to deciding how we are going to live our lives based upon how we think it is best to live our lives. We use our experience and our smarts to analyze the situation and then make a decision based upon the analysis. Examples of this are easy to find. You are looking for a parking spot at the mall to do some Christmas shopping and see an empty spot near the front. Knowing (using your smarts), based upon your experience, that such parking spots are to be cherished as they are rare, you take the spot. Easy decision. What to do for a career, who to marry, how many kids to have, well, those can be harder. The harder decisions are more likely to be turned over to God for some guidance. The problem is that not only should we be seeking God's will for hard decisions, we should be seeking God's will for everything.

Idolatry is elevating anything above God or God's will. I personally spend sometimes entire days not seeking God's will. By my actions, in my heart, I really behave as if I were serving myself. I elevate the priorities important to me. Me. Me. Me. An example of this for my life is my long pursuit of not getting fat. This was never a revelation from God through prayer. It was my own choosing. I suspect that is how most of us are eating: by our own choosing. Having been released from dietary law after the Apostolic Conference (Jerusalem Conference Acts 15), instead of giving thanks to God for easing the burden with eating, we just forgot about God altogether with how we are eating. Finish the prayer prior to the meal and then dig in.

And dig in we do. Each year the population gets fatter and fatter. I lived most of my life never once thinking of God's will in how I eat. I served only Karl's will. Serving my will instead of God's will sounds again a lot like Jonah running off to Tarshish. It also sounds a lot like idolatry. We are to seek the will of God in everything. This includes how we are fueling the temple of the Holy Spirit. Like it or not, you are a Temple. Or, "Do you not know that your bodies are temples of the Holy Spirit, who is in you, whom you have received from God? You are not your own; you were bought at a price. Therefore honor God with you bodies" (1 Corinthians 6:19-20).

You may not like to think of your body as a temple of God. But, it is a temple of God even if you are not treating it well, even if you are poisoning it with food, alcohol, or drugs. It is a temple of God even if you are the one running the show and using it to serve your own will instead of God's. It is a temple of God even if it is a mess. It is a temple of God even if you are a sinful idolater.

Alternatively, you may work very hard to have a hard and sexy temple. You may be proud of your temple. Your temple may be stacked, adorned with a hard ass, adorned with gold, adorned with perky breasts, adorned with shiny nails, adorned with a six pack, adorned with a tan, adorned with beautiful hair, adorned with expensive clothes. But, are you making your temple beautiful for God? Even if your temple is visually beautiful and healthy, if you are making it look good to serve your own will instead of God's will, you are still an idolater. You just happen to be idolizing yourself instead of your food. And you are just like me.

There is some really good news amongst all this mess. God loves us and has already forgiven us. God, knowing that we are not capable of keeping ourselves from idolatry, sent his only Son, as was prophesied in the scriptures. Jesus was killed on a cross for the forgiveness of all of our sins past, all of our sins present, and all of our sins future. We are fully forgiven for everything. God has placed all of the sin of man onto the shoulders of Jesus. Thank you, God. Thank you, Jesus.

As we have already been made holy and washed clean of all of our sin by the sacrifice of Jesus, there is no reason to try to work hard to earn anything from God. We cannot increase our standing with God by having a better temple. What we can do is be thankful. We are given grace, and grace is unmerited favor. We can be thankful even though we don't deserve it. We can be extra thankful *because* we don't deserve it. As a result of this gift of grace we may wish to express our gratitude by honoring God and honoring the sacrifice of Jesus. There are a few specific ways we are instructed to do this.

We are taught that if we sin, we are to repent and be baptized (Acts 2:38). We can confess our sin and ask forgiveness of God, but that is mostly for our psychological benefit because God has forgiven you even before your asking. So, assuming we are already forgiven, we are to repent. Baptism is a specific act of repentance. Repentance is a change in direction. We are to change our direction to be in line with the life of Jesus.

If you, like me, have been eating and exercising as a way to serve your own will, change direction. Begin to seek God's will for how you use your time. Seek God's will for how you beautify the temple of the Holy Spirit. Seek God's will for how you fuel his temple. The purpose of the law was to show that we, even with the best of intentions, cannot live our life in a way that is in line with the will of God on our own (Romans 3:20). Now that we have been released from the law, under the new covenant, that fact has not changed. Seek God's will for his temple.

Chapter: 18

Science Lesson #9 – The Sports Psychology of Eating

Jane is the best player on her basketball team. She knows it and the rest of the team does too. Early in the game Jane takes a shot, an easy one for her, and misses. One of the reasons Jane is the best is that she is a hard-working perfectionist. This miss of an easy shot is a real blow to Jane's psyche. She gets so upset that instead of trying for the rebound or running back on defense, she screams into the air and then hangs her head. Meanwhile the player Jane is guarding has run down the court unguarded and scores a lay-in at the other end.

Ron is a very good player. He is known for being physical and aggressive. Both of these are helpful traits, but on occasion Ron goes overboard and gets into fights on the playing surface. This results in his ejection and suspension for the next game.

Both Jane and Ron have taken traits that are good to extremes that are harmful. A lesson in sports psychology should help them both.

In medical school there is good training on psychiatry. The harms and merits of different anti-depressant medication and electroconvulsive therapy are part of a core curriculum. There is very little training on psychology. Perhaps that is because it is seen as a soft science. In sport there is very little need for Prozac, and Ritalin is illegal. Psychology however can mean the difference between first and last place. It was during my fellowship that I got my first real training in psychology. While it was sports psychology, the general principals apply to everyday life as well.

I will give the everyday example of my patient Heather. She has struggled with her weight since junior high school. Now, 20 years later, 40 diets later, hundreds of pounds lost and regained later, Heather is in my office with knee pain. Unfortunately for Heather, the extra weight she has been carrying around has caused her knee cartilage to wear out. She has osteoarthritis.

There were already incentives for Heather to lose weight. I did not go over these, I just stated that a part of a comprehensive treatment plan for knee arthritis at a young age was weight loss. When I saw Heather back in 2 weeks to recheck her knee, she had gained 3 pounds. This is not an uncommon outcome of counseling on weight loss, especially to someone who has not come to the office for that purpose. But why? Was it her way of saying, "Screw you Kaluza for telling me I need to lose weight!" A closer look at sports psychology will help.

There are many factors that influence behavior. But at a base level, there is simply seeking pleasure and avoiding pain. Heather had many reasons why losing weight would be pleasurable. Her knee would feel better, she would feel better about herself, she would have a better aesthetic, and she could eat with less guilt, etc. Place all of those on the "pro" list. So what would keep someone from doing what would lead to all of those benefits? What is on the "con" list? For that answer we have to look at Heather's past. She has tried to lose weight dozens, maybe hundreds of times in the past. Each time she has ultimately failed. Failure brings pain. The "con" list is short, but there is the answer, trying to lose weight causes pain. The best way to avoid this pain of failure is to not even try in the first place. You can't fail if you don't try. It is a bullet-proof pain avoidance strategy. It works wonderfully well in the setting of eating too much, drinking too much, drug use, tobacco use, and attempting to avoid any other creation that the heart is drawn toward.

In Heather's case, the hope of improvement in her knee, as well as the other benefits of weight loss, was not worth the risk. Remember that chance of failure in this present case, based upon prior data, is 100%. Those are hard odds to overcome. There are two ways to do it.

The first option is to find something in creation that will be worth more to Heather's heart than her pleasure of food and avoiding the pain of failing. In equation form it looks like this:

New Desire of Heart > (Pleasure From Food + Avoiding Pain From Failing)

At her first appointment I tried to place "avoiding pain from knee arthritis and knee replacement" as the new desire of her heart. It did not work. In the past, Heather sacrificed pleasure from food to lose weight for trips to sunny places where she would wear a swimsuit, for a high school reunion, and for her friend's wedding where she was the maid of honor. The problem as you may have already noted, is that all of those had ending times. When the time ended, so did the effort. And so did the weight loss.

We went a step deeper as well. We talked about her weight loss plan. Each plan that she has put into place in the past had been something that was not sustainable for her. Giving up sugar, not eating white things, eating only pickles on Tuesdays, not eating dinner, not eating lunch, fasting on Sundays, and being a vegan were all ideas tried and failed. Heather would have been able to tell me from the start that these were not sustainable food intake decisions. Each ultimately became too much work in the moment to maintain.

The next step was some fourth grade math. We looked at calorie intake, and measured her output (see science lessons #5 and #6). This proved what was already obvious. She had been eating more calories than she had been burning. When I asked why, she said, "I don't know." So I told her (science lesson #2, food is good like sex and drugs). While not realizing it on a conscious level, Heather eagerly admitted to using food as a comfort. We also discussed her fear of failure. At this point there was better insight into the problem, but there was still a problem.

If Heather had not had faith, I would have tried to make a compelling argument that being released from the oppressive guilt and anxiety about food was well worth the work to gain control over it. But Heather believes in God. I asked her if she had been serving God's will with how she was caring for the temple? This idea had never occurred to her. We did a quick refresher on the Gospel, how she is forgiven for this and all of her other sins because God loves her and Jesus died for her. Not only that, we are given the Holy Spirit to help us. I prayed for her to allow God and the Spirit to be a comfort and help to her, and to guide her in each moment as she is forced to choose how to care for the temple.

Heather lost weight, fifty pounds in all, and her knee is doing well enough. It was the Gospel that had the power to change her. Everything else had failed. The Gospel is the only thing that is not corruptible. Any other object of our desire that may compel us to change has the likelihood of rusting, dying, or sinning. When we have elevated a sinner (person), or part of creation (which will die or rust, melt or crumble) to a place of importance greater than God in our lives, we can be sure that we will be broken hearted. Only the incorruptible, only God, has the chance of filling our hearts in a way that we can trust with steadfastness.

Realizing that we have an idol hiding in our heart is a great first step. Ridding oneself of the idol may be hard or even impossible. Thank goodness then that God's love and forgiveness are endless. All that can be asked of us is that we try. If we are prayerfully seeking God's will and then trying to live out His will, we are then doing all which God could ask of us. If He requires more, we can trust it will be given unto us through the Holy Spirit. We will not be called to finish anything that we are not capable of doing. We will not be called to try anything that we are not capable of trying (1 Corinthians 10:13).

If you feel that God is calling you to care for His temple differently, then you can rest assured that you are fully capable of doing just that. God wants His will to be done.

Chapter: 19

A Word on Guilt

"*For godly sorrow produces a repentance that leads to salvation without regret, whereas worldly sorrow produces death.*" 2 Corinthians 7:10

Each of us has within us a little voice, or a feeling, which allows us to know right from wrong. It is called a conscience. A debate on the ethics of lying or stealing is interesting, but entirely unnecessary. We already know inside of ourselves that lying is wrong because our conscience tells us so. And it is not only you and me that has a conscience, it is everyone. This unifying fact of the human condition is one of the good arguments for a divine designer. From a Darwinian evolutionary perspective a conscience should be a hindrance and a disadvantage to passing on one's genetic material. Evolutionary theory is all about propagation of genes. You want to pass on your genes, and if you are good at it, then there will be more people like you in the future. If you are bad at it, then there will be fewer and fewer of you in the future and you will eventually become extinct.

I personally passed on my genetic material twice. If I had not had a conscience, it would have been much much much more than this. How then is a conscience explained? Why has this evolutionary disadvantage stuck around? It is because we have been created with a conscience. God has designed us with the ability to discern what is right and what is wrong. The apostle Paul states this in Romans chapter two speaking of the Gentile non-believers "For they show that the work of the law is written on their hearts, while their conscience also bears witness, and their conflicting thoughts accuse or even excuse them on that day when, according to my gospel, God judges the secrets of men by Christ Jesus." God has given us a conscience, a little voice that tells us righteousness from sin, and He has done so with a purpose.

God's purpose is conviction. If we are doing a sinful thing, God wishes us to know about it, and the conscience accomplishes this. God's plan with regard to our sin is really great and really simple. As He has already forgiven us, we are to give thanks for the undeserved grace of that forgiveness and for the undeserved sacrifice of Jesus that accomplished that forgiveness. Out of that thankful heart we are to repent. Repentance is a change in direction. If we have been sinning we have been walking away from Jesus and God. We are to turn around and run toward God. We are to change direction.

Note that repentance is not feeling sorry you got caught. It is not rationalizing why you were sinning. It is not blaming someone else. And it is definitely not feeling guilty about something for a long time. God's plan with regard to our sin is simple and beautiful and freeing. It should create unabashed joy within our hearts. But we sure do bugger it up.

Often the prick of the conscience will lead to focus on the self. We pridefully make it all about us. We feel guilty, and instead of repenting, we just wallow in self-focused guilt. This type of guilt and focus on self has derailed many an attempt at improving ourselves. Satan helps the earthly desires of our flesh to sin in the first place, and then he encourages us to languish, focused on ourselves, in our guilt. We may even think things like, "I don't deserve to be forgiven," or "God could not forgive me for that," or "I have done that sin so many times, I may as well not even try to stop," or "Even if God could forgive me, I can't forgive myself." Our adversary loves to trick us into focusing on our sin and ourselves when our focus should be on God. If we focus on God and His word, if we believe the gospel, then there is not a proper place for ongoing guilt. God has forgiven us. Jesus has already paid the price.

Because we have desires of the flesh, and because we live in a broken world, we will sin. We will be selfish in our relationships. We will choose to honor our own will instead of the will of God. We will be tempted by the adversary and succumb to his temptation. We will gossip. We will judge others. God, hating sin, will not like any of that behavior. But God, loving the sinner, sent Jesus so that He could justly have renewed perfect relationship with us as holy inheriting sons and daughters.

Out of that gift of God, and out of the sacrifice of Jesus, we are called not to guilt, but to repentance. We are not to be undone by our sins, failures, and shortcomings. Instead, we are to look to Jesus and try to align our lives with His.

If you are plagued by guilt, or if you use guilt as a means of controlling the behavior of someone else, it is time to stop. Take your eyes off of yourself and instead look to God for forgiveness and direction. The prick of the conscience then can be a quick tool that will lead to thanksgiving for the forgiveness given through the sacrifice of Jesus, and to repentance with the new direction given not by our will but by the will of God.

Continuing in our guilt and refusing to forgive ourselves or others is another form of idolatry. We are taught in scripture to forgive. Refusing to do so is simply another example of elevating our will above God's. If that causes a prick to the conscience, you know what to do.

Chapter: 20

Science Lesson # 10 – A Summary On a Healthy Temple:

"*What agreement has the temple of God with idols? For we are the temple of the living God; just as God said, 'I WILL DWELL IN THEM AND WALK AMONG THEM; AND I WILL BE THEIR GOD, AND THEY SHALL BE MY PEOPLE.*'" 2 Corinthians 6:16

"*May the favor of the Lord our God rest on us; establish the work of our hands for us- yes, establish the work of our hands.*" Psalm 90:17

The life of a professional athlete is glorious in some ways. Personally, I would be compelled by the opportunity to play a game for a paycheck. A big paycheck. The endless stream of well-wishers and girls sounds nice too. But it is not all fun games and pretty girls. There is a lot of hard work involved (much harder than most people work) and there is a toll taken on the body. And there is temptation.

Basketball all-star Charles Barkley's famous commercial of "I am not a role model" is great because it is both true and not true at the same time. It is easy to pick out areas of Sir Charles' life where he has behaved poorly as a role model. But he remains a role model, even if against his own will, because of his fame. With greater fame and greater wealth comes greater temptation. Solomon, the wisest man other than Jesus to ever have lived, could not resist the temptation of women, and it led to the downturn of an entire nation. There are an unfortunate number of professional athletes who have proven incapable of fairing any better than Solomon. But there are some counterexamples.

Of all of the professional athletes I have worked with, Futty Danso of the Portland Timbers is one that comes to mind when I think of the athletes I respect the most. Futty is Muslim. Each year he is called to fast during Ramadan. Despite the fact that this hurts him professionally (you try running 5 miles of wind sprints in Houston after fasting daily for a month), Futty does as he is called to do. If Futty is willing to sacrifice of himself like this, how much more should we be willing to sacrifice of ourselves given the grace of God bestowed unto us through Jesus?

This sacrifice of our selfish will to come into line with the will of God is different for each person. In my life it meant that I would exercise less. I was called to write this book, and I felt prodded to give up my exercise time as a way to make that happen. Book researching and writing took about 1000 hours. All 1000 of those hours came at the expense of exercise. My temple feels a little slower and weaker as a result, but I am stronger in spirit as a result of serving God's will. As the apostle Paul teaches in the book of

Romans, we are to try to live in the spirit, not in the flesh. So there is more to a healthy temple than strong muscles and soft skin.

For many people a healthier temple will mean some other sacrifice of self. It may mean more walking and less television. It may mean more bicycling and less eating. It may mean giving up alcohol. It may mean drinking a glass of red wine with dinner to help your cholesterol. As there is not a one size plan for all people. It will take prayer, reading scripture, and spiritual discernment to seek God's will. And it may require God's help to follow His will. Asking the Holy Spirit for assistance is not cheating, it is a help given to us by Jesus. Please take advantage.

Seeking and then honoring God's will for your body, mind, and spirit is point number one of a one point summary for this book. Nobody does this perfectly. Most of us do it poorly. Let's revisit some specifics that may be helpful in creating a healthy temple for God:

Exercise: Seek in exercise to honor God and not to honor the self. Know how many calories you are burning with your exercise by measuring your work rate. A heart rate monitor is a wonderful tool for measuring work rate. A clock is a poor measure of work rate. Ignore the government's instruction to exercise for a certain amount of time, and instead set goals of a specific amount of work.

Different people have different goals with exercise but everyone should be doing a combination of cardiovascular exercise and resistive exercise. For a marathon runner this would be 90% running and 10% resistance work. For a body builder this would be 90% resistance work and 10% cardio. Most of us fall somewhere in the middle.

Most people exercise less often than would be good for health. There are some people who exercise too much. In both settings there is some desire greater than God's will driving the decision making.

Eating: Seek in eating to honor God's will and not to honor the self. Know how many calories you are eating by counting them. Doing so for a short period of time will give tremendous insight into the more important half of the weight equation which is calorie intake. There are many wonderful applications for this online, on smarty phones and ipads, and in calorie counting books at the public library. If you do not know how many calories you are eating, you cannot know how to set goals for your work rate with exercise. If you do not know how many calories you are eating, I (or your doctor/nutritionist/etc) cannot as effectively help you make meaningful change in how you are eating.

There are four food groups: carbs, fat, protein, and alcohol. God created these as the only sources of calories for the human body. It is very helpful to know how many calories of each you are consuming. The low-fat diet that has been popular for "health" reasons in the past three decades may not be very healthy. Consuming any of the four food groups in anything other than moderation is a bad plan, especially if the unmoderated group is alcohol. Most people consume too much of the carbohydrate food group and the fat food group and not enough of the protein food group.

Trying to trick the system by eating artificial sweeteners, non-fat foods, low-fat foods, reduced-calorie foods, and sugar-free foods is always a bad idea. All of these foods will have food labels which will reveal the reason if you take the time to look. Even better, try to eat food which was available to us in the Garden of Eden (which does not have a label).

For the carbohydrates that we do eat, we should strive to make them last longer than our insulin. This requires eating foods that are low glycemic index which are digested slowly. The low glycemic index foods will have a positive impact on energy levels and will keep insulin levels lower. Lower insulin means less growing because insulin is a growth factor. If you are not growing taller, you can guess the only other way to grow as an adult.

I try to make it simple for my patients when they make food choices. I provide a list of foods to eat and foods to avoid. I try to make the eat list longer than the avoid list so people can concentrate on the positive. Studies have shown the following to be healthful: fish, nuts and seeds, red wine, fruits and vegetables, olive oil, and dark chocolate (see the afterward B at the end of the book for more information on fish, red wine, and whole grains). Studies have shown the following foods to be harmful: artificial sweeteners, corn syrup, refined grains, and trans-fats (hydrogenated oils and almost everything deep-fried). I suggest eating the foods that will provide good fuel for your temple and avoiding the harmful foods. But, my input is not important. Ask God His will for your care of the temple. God's will be done.

Pleasure: In seeking pleasure honor God's will, not your own will. Know the sources of pleasure in your life. These may include food, sex, exercise, love, drugs, music, art, and laughter. Trying to fill your heart's desire for pleasure with just drugs, just sex, just food, or just laughing will not work. It will cause problems. Consoling yourself with food because you are not happy will only lead to future unhappiness. Consoling yourself with alcohol will only lead to future unhappiness. Pleasuring yourself with drugs or alcohol is dangerous because of addiction. Addiction is continued use despite adverse consequences which requires elevating something above God and His will. It is idolatry.

We should be plenty pleased simply with God's undeserved grace given to us in the form of our savior Jesus and with the joys of creation. We should serve the Creator and not the creation. In times when we serve the creation, including our created selves, we should repent and move in a new direction. We can know that the new direction is correct if it is bringing us closer to Jesus. God helps us to do this by giving us a moral conscience.

Cheating: Artificial sweeteners, low fat food, low calorie foods, weight loss pills, potions, and shots, and all other forms of trying to circumvent a simple plan of eating well and exercising do not work. Placing your hope in any of these products is likely a path to failure. If you need something to place your hope in, place it in Jesus. Jesus actually lived and actually died for you. Faith in Him produces hope, joy, and peace.

Chapter: 21

A Benediction

"The Spirit and the bride say "Come!" And let him who hears say, "Come!" Whoever is thirsty, let him come; and whoever wishes, let him take the free gift of the water of life... "Yes, I am coming soon." Amen. Come, Lord Jesus. The grace of the Lord Jesus be with God's people. Amen." Revelation 22:17-18

It has been my goal in writing this book to proclaim the good news available to all people of the death and resurrection of Jesus for the forgiveness of our sins. It has been my goal to prove that we are all in need of such forgiveness due to our sinful idolatry in serving the creation, including our created selves, instead of the Creator. It has been my goal to have this stir repentance in how we are caring for the temple of the Holy Spirit. Take good care of yourself for you are not your own, you are a temple of God. I pray that God will prick our conscience and lead us on the right path of repentance where peace and joy await, in the name of Jesus who lives and reigns forever and ever. Amen.

About the Author:

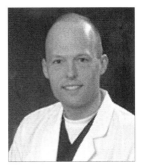

I spent years of my life mocking the faithful and scorning the hypocritical self-righteous judgment of organized religion. While I can't undo the damage I caused to other's trust in God, I will spend the rest of my life as a living testimony to the power of God to change lives. I hope that my story and my knowledge about food, exercise, and nutrition are able to inspire hope, joy, and peace as we care for the temple of the Holy Spirit.

Afterward A:

A list of artificial and non-nutritive sweeteners all of which have the potential to cause the diet soda/artificial sweetener effect:

- sucralose (Splenda)
- aspartame (NutraSweet, Equal)
- acesulfame potassium (Nutrinova)
- cyclamate
- dulcin
- glucin
- neotame
- saccharin
- xylitol
- sorbitol
- mannitol
- maltitol
- lactitol
- isomalt
- inulin
- glycerol
- erythritol
- curculin
- stevia - I get a lot "it is natural" arguments when people think they should be eating stevia. My reply is that cocaine is a natural plant too, that does not mean it is good for you. (From the FDA website: "FDA has not permitted the use of whole-leaf Stevia or crude Stevia extracts because these substances have not been approved for use as a

food additive. FDA does not consider their use in food to be GRAS (generally regarded as safe) in light of reports in the literature that raise concerns about the use of these substances. Among these concerns are control of blood sugar and effects on the reproductive, cardiovascular, and renal systems.").

Afterward B:

There are aspects of looking at what we know of how Jesus ate that will also be good for us in the present day. I am not speaking of a return to eating under the law or to Old Testament rules. There have been a couple of books written in this vein suggesting that eating a sprouted grain Ezekiel diet or a Kosher diet will be good for our health because that is what Jesus, a Jew, would have eaten. The problem with that line of thinking is that we are specifically instructed in the New Testament that we have been released from the burden of the law. Therefore, that argument, being specifically contrary to scriptural teaching, holds no water. Perhaps though, there are aspects of how Jesus ate that can provide some insight into righteous eating.

Jesus ate with other people. There are no examples in scripture of Jesus eating alone. Often when we eat alone we eat poorly. This can be avoided by eating with others. In addition to avoiding something harmful, eating with others gives opportunity for building and bolstering, encouraging and exhorting, and sharing our lives. Shared meals are often the most joyous and memorable sources of pleasure in our lives. Make a point of eating with others.

Jesus ate fish. Fish is very good for you. People who eat more fish have higher intelligence. People who eat more fish have lower cholesterol. People who eat more fish have fewer heart attacks and strokes. People who eat more fish have larger penises. Well, that last one is not proven, but it may be true. The only down side to eating fish is a concern regarding mercury. Mercury is a heavy metal that can cause brain and nerve problems. Because of pollution fish can have high mercury levels. This creates a tension between known benefit and potential harm.

Many women have given up eating fish while pregnant out of a concern for the potential harm to the baby. It is my recommendation to eat fish frequently even while pregnant. The benefit simply outweighs the risk. The Seychelles Child Development Study offers proof. In the Seychelles, which is a group of islands in the Indian Ocean, 85% of people eat fish daily (study average was 12 servings per week). Due to this high fish consumption there is a higher risk of mercury toxicity as ocean fishes around the world contain about the same levels of mercury. Additionally, in the Seychelles, there is no other source of mercury, meaning that the mercury effects of fish can be studied specifically. There was no harm found from high fish consumption in the Seychelles even though people's mercury levels were up to 20 times higher than those seen in the USA.

That said, it does make sense to me to attempt to limit mercury intake. This means eating smaller fish. Big fish eat small fish and concentrate the mercury. The further up the seafood chain you move, the higher the mercury level. It also means that wild fish are likely preferable to farm-raised fish. Most studies on mercury content have shown a consistently higher level in farm-raised fish compared to wild fish. So eat lots of wild fish, just like Jesus. In fact, Jesus liked fish so much he kept eating it even after he was raised from the dead.

Jesus also drank wine. This fact is somehow very controversial. As if Jesus, being good and all, would not drink something bad like wine. Let's start with what we can know from science: Red wine, consumed in moderation defined as two glasses per day or less for men and one glass or less per day for women, has many known health benefits. Red wine decreases the risk of all forms of cardiovascular disease including heart attacks and strokes. Red wine decreases the risk of prostate cancer. Red wine decreases the risk of breast cancer. Red wine decreases the risk of lung cancer. Red wine is good for cholesterol. Red wine decreases the risk of dementia. Red wine decreases the risk of diabetes. Diabetic who drink red wine have lower blood sugars. People who drink red wine in moderation report being happier that people who drink to excess or abstain. People who drink red wine get fewer colds. And red wine drinkers live longer.

The myth that you can get the same benefits from consuming an extract of the grape skin called reservatrol has been disproven by Washington University researchers in data released in the journal *Cell Metabolism* in 2012. Nor has the benefit of red wine been shown to be present when drinking unfermented grape juice. Wine and beer qualitatively and quantitatively change fibrinogen, a clotting factor in the blood. Reservatrol and grape juice have not been shown to do this. Next, let's look at scripture.

In John 2, Jesus' first miracle was to make wine for revelers at the wedding at Cana. This was not only wine (Greek = *oinos*), it was good wine (*kailon onion*), a term used for fermented wine found elsewhere in the New Testament. Jesus, being sinless, would not have produced an inherently sinful product.

We also know Jesus had the reputation of a glutton and a drunkard among his accusers. You do not get such a reputation without eating and drinking. Luke and Matthew have parallel verses regarding Jesus speaking on this point. "For John (the Baptist) came neither eating nor drinking, and they say, 'He has a demon.' The Son of Man came eating and drinking, and they say, 'Here is a glutton and a drunkard, a friend of tax collectors and sinners.' But wisdom is proved right by her deeds." We can thus see Jesus both making wine and drinking wine in scripture, and then there is the last supper.

Jesus not only drank wine himself, he commanded us to drink wine in memory of Him. At the last supper he raised the Passover cup, filled with Passover wine, and said in Matthew 26, Mark 14, and Luke 22 to drink of it in his memory, "For I tell you that from now on I will not drink of the fruit of the vine until the kingdom of God comes...This cup that is poured out for you is the covenant in my blood." (The Passover celebration takes place in the spring. Grape harvest takes place in the fall. Any grape juice still around 6 months after harvest with no pasteurization and no refrigeration will be fermented whether you want it to be or not.)

Therefore, there are reasons that one may want to drink wine. But there are many reasons not to drink wine as well. Some people think that it is sinful to drink alcohol. The apostle Paul teaches in 1 Corinthians 8:13 that when it comes to a controversial food, we are to avoid it if others think that it is sinful so as not to cause them discomfort. We are warned many times in scripture against drunkenness. Wine can cause drunkenness which is sinful.

If wine turns you into an asshole or a slut it should be avoided. Some people cannot drink wine without elevating it above God's will. One sip will lead to the total inability of their flesh to not take the next sip. And then another, and another, and another, leading to drunkenness. Alcoholism, which may affect as many as one person in ten, has both genetic and environmental causes. Alcoholism is continued use of alcohol despite adverse consequences. But even those of us who are not alcoholics can use wine in a way that is sinful, even if we avoid drunkenness. If we place the act or desire of our will above the will of God, then we have made the wine (again a product of creation) into an idol. If I get home from work after a hard day and it is God's will for me to play with my kids, and instead I head to the fridge for a beer, I have just been guilty not of drunkenness, but idolatry.

Wine should therefore be consumed as a good and healthy gift of God only in ways that are not idolatrous and do not lead to drunkenness. One glass or less per day for women, and two glasses per day or less for men (men have a greater ability to metabolize alcohol). Like any other gift of creation, if it is leading to sin, if it cannot be enjoyed in a fashion that is aligned with God's will, then it should be avoided.

Another notable feature of how Jesus ate can be seen with bread. Jesus produced bread as one of his miracles. In the gospel of Luke (22:19) He instructed us to think of him as we break and eat bread. "And he took bread, gave thanks and broke it, and gave it to them, saying, 'This is my body given for you; do this in remembrance of me.'"

Jesus was not eating super spongy melt in your mouth white bread. He was eating whole grain bread. Whole grains are a good source of low glycemic index carbohydrate, protein, and fiber. Eating whole grains decreases the risk of diabetes, stroke, heart disease, obesity, colon cancer, high blood pressure, and gum and tooth disease. This all sounds great, but it is relative to eating refined grains. Please refer to the marketing trickery in chapter 13 regarding the traps of finding foods that are actually whole grain. The whole grain studies can also be read in reverse showing that eating refined grains increases the risk of obesity, diabetes, heart disease, and gum disease. Stick with 100% whole grain foods, just like Jesus.

16411920R00089

Made in the USA
San Bernardino, CA
03 November 2014